国家中医药管理局国际合作项目"中国–老挝中医药中心"项目
云南省商务厅"云南省中医药服务出口基地"项目

云南本草图鉴

郑　进　　左媛媛　主编

U0200134

学苑出版社

图书在版编目（CIP）数据

云南本草图鉴/郑进，左媛媛主编．－－北京：学苑出版社，2025.1．－－ISBN 978－7－5077－7041－4

Ⅰ．R281.474－64

中国国家版本馆 CIP 数据核字第 20244GQ403 号

责任编辑：黄小龙
出版发行：学苑出版社
社　　　址：北京市丰台区南方庄 2 号院 1 号楼
邮政编码：100079
网　　　址：www.book001.com
电子邮箱：xueyuanpress@163.com
联系电话：010－67601101（营销部）、010－67603091（总编室）
印　刷　厂：北京兰星球彩色印刷有限公司
开本尺寸：710 mm×1000 mm　1/16
印　　　张：10
字　　　数：159 千字
版　　　次：2025 年 1 月第 1 版
印　　　次：2025 年 1 月第 1 次印刷
定　　　价：88.00 元

编 委 会

主　编　郑　进　左媛媛

副主编　孙永林　王　璟　王进进

编　委　(按姓氏笔画排序)

付现春　刘仲书　刘楚婷　严　瑶　李玉卿

李海涛　吴　非　何开仁　张　慧　张大宝

解宇环

主　译　赵少钦

插　画　钱仕翠

前　言

徐霞客游历云南时，曾赞誉云南："桃花流水，不出人间，云影苔痕，自成岁月。"很多到过云南的人都说，云南是个被上天眷顾的地方，好山、好水、好气候。其独特的地理位置和多样的气候条件成就了"植物王国"的美誉，更有数千种中草药植物在这里繁衍生息。

云南自古以来就是中草药的重要产地和交流中心，这里有着悠久的中药文化传统，许多中药的研究和应用经验代代相传。世代居住在这里的各族人民，就地取材，从高山峻岭到河谷平原，从热带雨林到高山草甸，通过千百年来的经验总结，认药、用药、食药，形成了独具特色而又疗效显著的传统医药治疗方法，也筛选出了种类丰富、疗效确切的天然植物药。

在云南，人们与植物、与动物、与自然的关系是密切的，很多药用植物就长在房前屋后、街角路边。从高山上热烈绽放的杜鹃花，到热带雨林中枝枝蔓蔓的藤本植物，那高耸挺拔的南方嘉木中有药，那绿意盎然的草本植物中有药，枝头的花里有药，路边的草里也有药……

本书选取了云南中医药、民族医药中颇具代表性的，也是田间地头最为常见的107种中草药，按视频拍摄的时间先后排序，从植物科属、中药性味、归经和功效等方面，向大家科普云南常见药物、道地药物。希望读者能先了解身边最为常见的花花草草，再由植物而了解中医药、健康保健，从知晓植物知识到认识在地自然。当书中之药与眼前之草不期而遇时，进一步发现云南之美、植物之美、草药之美！

全书中草药配有手绘的彩图，读者扫描书中的二维码，还可观看视频，能直观地看到此味中药的生长环境、状态，又能听到相应的科普讲解。中英双语的文字解读，便于本书海外传播，更可以作为中小学生的中医药文化、自然科普读物。

书中视频原声解读均来自本书主编之一郑进教授。他在三年多的时间里，在下乡义诊的路上、上山采药的路上，坚持不懈地拍摄、记录着这些云南人身边常见的、少数民族世代常用的花花草草。视频剪辑和加字幕的工作也由郑教授完成。因为原始视频丢失，所以视频中的双重字幕和文字错误等无法修改，请读者谅解。以后有机会再替换有误的视频。在拍摄记录的过程中，还得到了中国医学科学院药用植物研究所李海涛教授、云县中医医院张慧主任医师、德宏何开仁主任医师、蒙自中医医院刘仲书医生等同道的大力支持，这些朋友积极提供视频素材和用药经验。本书选取的中草药只是云贵高原丰富药用植物中的一小部分，更多有用、有趣的"路边草药"还等待着各位同道不断发掘整理，书中错漏之处也希望能得到广大读者的批评和指正。

最后，团队所有的努力都是为了让广大中医药爱好者们体验一次沉浸式的阅读，感受云南这个充满生机和活力的"植物王国"，发现云南除了山美、水美、人美之外，还有很多药用价值较高的中草药，以及与之相生相伴的博大精深的传统医药文化。

编者

甲辰年（2024）仲春

目　录

1. 黄连木 *Pistacia chinensis* Bunge

黄连木，漆树科，黄连木属。这种高大落叶乔木在云南有很多，在城市和乡镇随处可见，在云南又称其为黄连树、茶树。在秋冬落叶之前它的叶子变黄变红，特别漂亮。云南本地人，常把它的嫩叶摘回家焯水当菜吃，有一股清香的味道，因此，云南有的地方也把它叫作清香木。黄连木也是我们身边的一味草药，它在我国的分布很广，它的叶、芽、根、树干都可以入药，其味苦涩，性寒，具有清热、生津、解毒和利湿的功效。

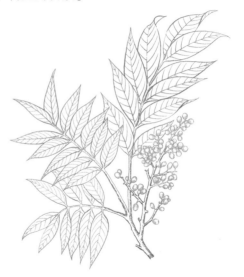

Pistacia chinensis Bunge is tall and big deciduous tree of Anacardiaceae and *Pistacia chinensis* Bunge family. They can be easily found in the villages, towns and cities in Yunnan province. They are also called Huanglianshu or tea tree in Yunnan. Their leaves are extremely beautiful when they turn into yellow and red in autumn and winter. People often collect their tender leaves and take them as vegetables after being blanched them briefly in boiled water, thus they are obtained another name of Qingxiangmu due to their fragrant flavor. *Pistacia chinensis* Bunge is also a kind of herbs around us, which is widely distributed in China, its leaves, buds, roots, stems and bark can be used as medicine. It tastes bitter with cold property and it can clear heat, generate fluid, detoxificate and remove dampness.

2. 丽春花(虞美人) *Papaver rhoeas* L.

在春暖花开的季节里，虞美人格外引人注目，它给城市带来色彩和生机。虞美人不仅作为花卉供人欣赏，它还是我们身边的一味草药。这种原产于欧洲的花卉来到我国以后，也被我们的祖先发现了它的药用价值，明代著名医家李时珍就在他的《本草纲目》中记载了作为中药使用的虞美人。虞美人的中药名叫丽春花，它和罂粟同科同属，全草都可入药，其味苦涩，性微寒，有毒，具有镇咳镇痛和止泻的功效。

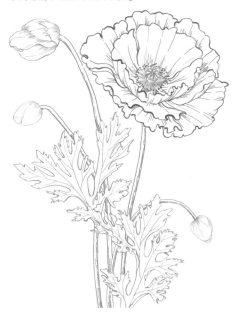

Papaver rhoeas L. is particularly eye-catching during the spring season for its color and vitality. It is not only a flower for people to appreciate, but also a kind of herb around us. Our ancestors found its medicinal value that native to Europe after it had been introduced to China, Li Shizhen, a famous doctor in the Ming Dynasty, recorded the use of *Papaver rhoeas* L. as traditional Chinese medicine in his *Compendium of Materia Medica* that it belongs to the same family and genus of poppy and its flowers and fruits can be used as medicine. It tastes bitter with minor cold property, and it can soothe cough, relieve pain and stop diarrhea.

临床上可用它来治疗咳嗽日久、偏头痛、腹痛，以及痢疾。据《中国藏药》记载，它的花还可以治疗瘀血腹痛，以及邪热妄行导致的身痛。

It can be used to treat chronic cough, hemicrania, stomachache and dysentery clinically. Its flowers can also cure abdominal pain blood stasis, as well as the body pain caused by evil heat according to *Chinese Tibetan Medicine*.

3. 芦荟

Aloe vera（L.）Burm. f.

说起"芦荟"，很多人知道它是美容佳品，但却很少有人知道它也是一味中药。芦荟，阿福花科，芦荟属。它的汁液经过干燥浓缩以后就可以入药，其味苦，性寒，具有泻下清肝和杀虫的功效。芦荟虽然无毒，但是体质虚寒的患者以及孕妇是不建议使用的。芦荟的现代药理研究特别多，首先，它的抗肿瘤作用是明确的，相关的研究文献也特别多。此外，芦荟还有明显的免疫调节和抗衰老的作用。

When talking about *Aloe vera*, many people may know that it is an ideal cosmetic product, but few people know that it is also a traditional Chinese medicine, it belongs to aloe family and genus. Its juice can be used as medicine for purging the liver and killing the insects after being dried and concentrated. It tastes bitter with cold property. Although aloe vera is non-toxic, patients with physical deficiency and cold constitution as well as pregnant women are not suggested to use. There are many pharmacological researches and numerous literatures on *Aloe vera*, which furtherly confirmed its anti-cancer effect, furthermore, it also has obvious effects of regulating immunomodulatory and anti-aging.

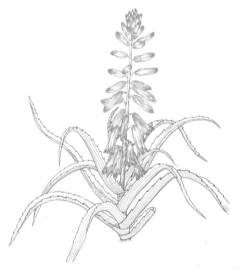

4. 素馨花

Jasminum grandiflorum Linn.

素馨花，为木犀科茉莉花属植物，分布于四川、贵州、云南等地。盛开于春分时节的素馨花，其花朵不仅赏心悦目，香味沁人心脾，还是我们身边一味疗效确切的中草药。

Jasminum grandiflorum Linn. is the whole plant of the Jasmine family and Oleaceae, and it is mainly distributed in Sichuan, Guizhou and Yunnan provinces. It often blooms during the Vernal Equinox and its flowers are not only delightful in appearance with refreshing fragrance, but also an effective herbal medicine around us.

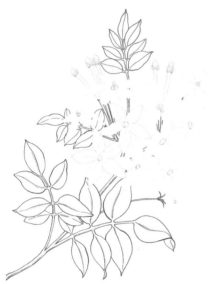

李时珍在他的《本草纲目》当中就介绍了素馨花的药用价值，这种木犀科攀缘灌木植物在我国的分布很广，《中华本草》介绍的素馨花的入药部位就是其花蕾。

Li Shizhen, a famous doctor in the Ming Dynasty, illustrated the medicinal value of *Jasminum grandiflorum* Linn in his *Compendium of Materia Medica*. It was widely distributed in China. *Chinese Materia Medica* mentioned that the buds of *Jasminum grandiflorum* Linn were used as medicine.

春天，将素馨花花蕾采摘后，隔水蒸，取出晒干以后就可以入药。《全国中草药汇编》则把素馨花的入药部位扩大到全株。素馨花，味苦，性平，归肝经。具有行气止痛，调经，清热散结之功效。常用于胃痛、肝炎、乳腺炎、月经不调、痛经、带下、口腔炎、睾丸炎、皮肤瘙痒、淋巴结结核。

The buds of *Jasminum grandiflorum* Linn. can be used as medicine after being collected, steamed and dried in the sun in spring. While *the National Collec-*

tion of Chinese Herbal Medicine expanded the medicinal parts of Jasminum grandiflorum Linn to the whole parts. It belongs to liver meridian and tastes bitter with mild property, it has the effect of regulating Qi and relieving pain, menstrual regulation, clearing heat and removing stasis. It can be used to treat stomachache, hepatitis, mastitis, irregular menstruation, dysmenorrhea, leukorrhagia, stomatitis, orchitis, skin pruritus and tuberculous lymphadenitis.

5. 癣草（南欧大戟）   *Euphorbia peplus* L.

　　在城市的街边、墙角、花坛和草地，到处可以见到这种野草，折断它的枝叶可以流出乳白色的浆液，这就是原产于地中海一带的大戟科大戟属植物南欧大戟。它主要分布在澳大利亚、美洲、亚洲，以及中国台湾、香港、福建、广西、云南、广东等地。

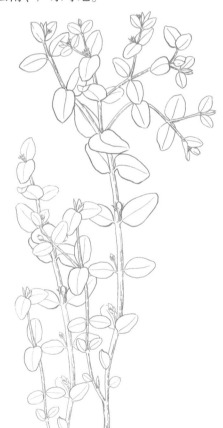

This kind of weed can be found everywhere in the corner of the flower beds and grasslands on the roadsides, and a milky slurry will be discharged when break off its branches and leaves, which is the Euphorbia peplus that native to the Mediterranean and mainly distributed in Australia, America, Asia and Taiwan, Hong Kong, Fujian, Guangxi, Yunnan and Guangdong.

　　南欧大戟来到中国以后逐渐变成我们身边的一味草药，它的中药名叫癣草，顾名思义它是治疗癣疮的一味草药。它的地上部分或者白色浆液是中医的入药部位，其味苦，性寒，有毒。外用于癣疮，有杀虫、解毒的功效。

Euphorbia peplus has gradually become a herb around us after it was introduced to China, it is called ringworm grass in traditional Chinese medicine and it can be used for treating ringworm sores just as its name implies. Its above-ground parts or white liquid are used as medicine, and it tastes bitter and has poison with cold property. It can be used externally for curing ringworm sores and it has the effects of killing insects and detoxification.

需要说明的是这是一味有毒中药，只能外用，如果误食以后可能引起中毒，轻者可以出现腹痛、呕吐，重者可以出现胃穿孔或者是肝肾功能的损害。孕妇、哺乳期妇女及过敏体质的人是不能使用的。

Attention should be paid to that Euphorbia peplus is a toxic herbal medicine and it can be used externally only. If someone takes it by mistake, it will cause poisoning symptoms, such as abdominal pain and vomiting for mild cases and stomach perforation or liver and kidney function damage for severe cases. Pregnant and lactating women as well as people with allergic constitution are not allowed to use it.

6. 小飞蓬

Erigeron canadensis L.

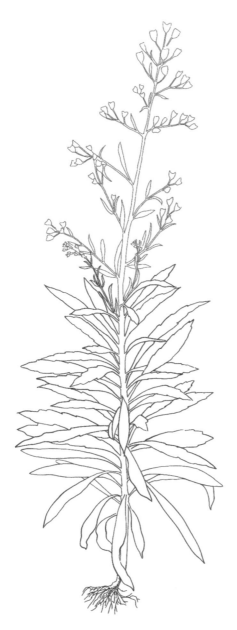

小飞蓬这种菊科一年生或者两年生草本植物，在我国的分布很广，路边、山坡、草地，以及城市的各个角落，到处可见。小飞蓬全草可以入药，其味微苦、辛，性凉，具有清热利湿、散瘀消肿的功效。

Erigeron canadensis L. is an annual or biennial herbaceous plant of the composite family. It is widely distributed in China, and it can be found on the roadside, hillside, grassland and every corner of the city. Its whole plant can be used as medicine, it tastes slightly bitter and pungent with cold property. It has the effects of clearing heat and dampness, dispersing blood stasis and detumescence.

对小飞蓬的现代药理研究特别多。首先，其抗菌消炎作用是明确的，小飞蓬中所含的香草酸和丁香酸是抗菌的有效成分。现代研究还证明：小飞蓬总黄酮水溶性部分，还有扩张冠状动脉的作用，其水提取物还有轻微的、短暂的降血压作用，这与小飞蓬抑制心脏、增加呼吸幅度有关。除了抗菌和对心血管系统有作用，小飞蓬还有明显的抗病毒活性的作用。

There are many modern pharmacological researches on Erigeron canadensis L., its antibacterial and anti-inflammatory effect is unequivocal, and the vanillic acid and syringic acid contained in it are the effective antibacterial components. Modern research also proves that the water-soluble part of its total flavones also has the effect of dilating coronary arteries and its water extract also has a slight and transient hypotensive effect, which is associated with its function of suppressing the heart and increasing breathing rate. In addition to being antibacterial and having an effect on the cardiovascular system, it also has significant function of antiviral activity.

小飞蓬适应性强，分布广，资源十分丰富，以上现代药理研究也从不同方面提示了我们：小飞蓬的药用价值非常高，是我们身边一味值得深入开发和研究的中草药。

Erigeron canadensis L. has a strong adaptability, wide range of distributionwith abundant resources. The above modern pharmacological studies also show us from different perspectives that Erigeron canadensis L. has a comparatively high medicinal value and it is also a Chinese herbal medicine worth further developing and researching.

7. 蛇莓

Duchesnea indica（Andr.）Focke in Engler & Prantl

这种山坡草地，河边、阴湿地，常见的小红果，就是可作为中药的蛇莓。蛇莓在我国的分布很广，除了东北以外几乎全国都有分布，这种蔷薇科多年生草本植物的全草都是中医的入药部位。其味甘、苦，性寒，具有清热解毒、散瘀消肿和凉血止血的功效。

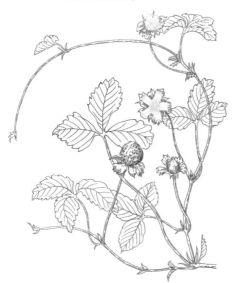

The common small red fruit on hillside grassland, river side, wet and dampground is the traditional Chinese medicine called *Duchesnea indica* (Andr.) Focke. It is widely distributed in almost all over the country except northeast China, the whole herb of this perennial plant of rose family can be used as medicine. It tastes sweet and bitter with cold property, and it has the effects of clearing heat, removing toxicity, eliminating stasis to subdue swelling and cooling blood for hemostasis.

蛇莓作为中药使用，最早见于陶弘景的《名医别录》，其名称也来源于《名医别录》。民间传说蛇莓有毒，关于其毒性问题，较为权威的说明是刘氏标等学者在 2009 年第 3 期《营养学报》中发表的一篇文章。他们在对小鼠进行急性毒性试验以后发现，小鼠无一死亡，而且测不出半数致死量，所以根据食品毒理学急性毒性分级标准，表明蛇莓果实是无毒的。

The use of *Duchesnea indica*(Andr.) Focke as traditional Chinese medicine was first recorded in *Supplementary Records of Famous Physicians* by Tao Hongjing, and its name was also originated from it. A folk legend once said that the Duchesneaindicaa(Andr.) FFockeand is poisonous, in order to test its toxicity, Liu Shibiao and other scholars made an authoritative explanation by performing acute toxicity tests on rats and publishing an article in the 3rd issue of *Chinese Journal of Nutrition* in 2009, finding that none of the mice died. Therefore, *Duchesnea indica*(Andr.) Focke is non-toxic.

8. 蒲公英

Taraxacum mongolicum Hand. -Mazz.

春天一到，遍地的这种小黄花特别引人注目，这就是著名的中药蒲公英。这种菊科一年生草本植物在我国的分布非常广泛，东南西北到处可见，蒲公英有很多名字：黄花地丁、地丁、婆婆丁、奶汁草、奶浆草。蒲公英全草都可以入药，其味苦、甘，性寒，具有清热解毒、消痈散结的功效。蒲公英既可以内服也可以外用，临床上可以用它来治疗乳痈、肺痈、肠痈（阑尾炎）、痄腮、疔毒疮疖、目赤肿痛、感冒发热、咳嗽、咽喉肿痛、肠炎、胃炎、痢疾、肝炎、胆囊炎、尿路感染和虫蛇咬伤。

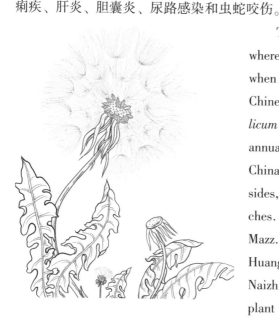

The small yellow flowers everywhere are particularly eye-catching when spring comes, this is the famous Chinese medicine *Taraxacum mongolicum* Hand. -Mazz. . This Compositae annual herb is widely distributed in China, it can be seen on the roadsides, hillsides, grassland and ditches. *Taraxacum mongolicum* Hand. -Mazz. has many names, such as Huanghuadiding, Diding, Popoding, Naizhicao and Naijiangcao. Its whole plant can be used as medicine, it tastes bitter and sweet with cold property, and it has the effects of clearing heat, removing toxicity, eliminating carbuncle and removing stasis. It can be taken internally or used exteriorly, and it is mainly used clinically to treat mastitis, pulmonary carbuncle, intestinal carbuncle (appendicitis), mumps, furunculosis, sore red swollen eyes, cold and fever, cough, sore throat, enteritis, gastritis, dysentery, hepatitis, cholecystitis, urinary tract infection as well as snake and insect bites.

由于蒲公英味苦性寒，所以不建议阳虚外寒和脾胃虚弱的患者使用。蒲公英的现代药理研究特别多，目前绝大部分集中在抗菌研究方面。现代药理研究还证明了蒲公英具有利胆保肝和抗胃损伤的作用，有学者研究证明蒲公英煎剂能够明显减轻大鼠应激反应所导致的胃黏膜损伤，使溃疡的发生率显著下降。蒲公英与中药党参和川芎配合使用后的抗溃疡作用更强。研究还进一步证明：三味药配伍使用后，能够明显地改善胃肠道血液的流变性和微循环，从而增加胃的血供。

It is not recommended for patients with Yang deficiency and external cold, spleen and stomach weakness to use it due to its cold property with bitterness in taste. There are many modern pharmacological studies on it, and most of them focus on antibacterial research. And the modern pharmacological researches also prove that the decoction of Taraxacum mongolicum Hand. Mazz. can obviously reduce the gastric mucosal damage caused by stress reaction in rats and significantly reduce the occurrence rate of ulcer. Furthermore, the combination of Taraxacum mongolicum Hand. Mazz. with Dangshen and Chuanxiong can have a stronger anti-ulcer effect. The researches also certify that the compatibility of the three medicines can significantly improve the rheology and microcirculation of gastrointestinal blood by increasing the blood supply to the stomach.

除此之外，还有很多蒲公英抗肿瘤、调节性激素、改善高胆固醇血症、促进乳汁分泌、利尿、调节动脉的舒张与收缩等很多方面作用的研究。蒲公英这棵路边小小的药草，是值得我们高度关注的一味中药材。

In addition, there are also many researches on the role of Taraxacum mongolicum Hand. Mazz. on anti-cancer, regulating hormones, improving hypercholesterolemia, promoting breast milk secretion, diuresis, regulating arterial diastole and contraction, etc., Taraxacum mongolicum Hand. Mazz., although it is a small roadside herbal medicine, it is a medicine that deserves our high attention.

9. 野艾蒿

Artemisia lavandulifolia DL.

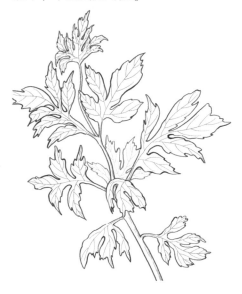

野艾蒿这种草药，在很长一段时间被人们当作野草，也有民间医生会用这种草作为刀伤止血或者是外伤止血的草药。

这种野草实际上就是菊科蒿属的多年生草本植物，也叫野艾，在我国的分布很广，从南到北、从东到西，到处都有，路边山坡、灌木、草丛到处可见。

Artemisia lavandulifolia DL. was regarded as a weed by people for a long time, and some folk doctors adopted this herb to stop bleeding for knife wounds or trauma. This weed is actually a perennial herb of the Artemisia family, also known as Ye'ai (mugwort), it is widely distributed in China and it is can be seen everywhere, such as the roadside slopes, shrubs and bushes.

野艾蒿也可以作为艾的代用品，其地上部分可以入药，味苦、辛，性温，具有理气行血、散寒调经、安胎、祛风除湿和消肿止血的功效，临床可以用它来治疗风寒感冒、头痛、心腹冷痛、泄泻、久痢、吐血、衄血、大便下血、月经不调、崩漏、带下、胎动不安、皮肤痈疮和疥癣。内服可以煎汤、捣汁、入丸散，外用可以捣敷或者煎汤洗，也可炒热温熨，还可以捣绒作为艾柱使用。

Artemisia lavandulifolia DL. can be used as a substitute for moxa, its above ground parts have bitter and pungent taste with warm property, and they can be used as medicine. It has the effects of regulating Qi and blood, dispelling cold and regulating menstruation, preventing miscarriage, dispelling wind and removing dampness, reducing swelling and hemostasis. It can be used clinically to treat cold, headache, cold pain in the heart and abdomen, diarrhea, chronic dysentery, vomiting blood, epistaxis, blood in stool, irregular menstruation, discontinuous leakage, abnormal vaginal discharge, fetal irritability, skin abscess and scabies. It can be decocted and taken internally, or mashed it into juice to make pill powder, or mashed it to apply or boiled to wash for external use. In addition, it can also be stir-fried hot for medicated compress or pounded into mugwort spunk and used as moxa cone.

10. 冬葵

Malva verticilata var. Crispa L.

只要你留意城市的角落、路边、花坛，到处可以见到这种野草，它可是我们身边的一味好药。冬葵是锦葵科锦葵属两年生草本植物，也有人叫它土黄芪，或者也叫它野葵，它也可以作为蔬菜食用，它的蔬菜名叫冬寒菜或者冬苋菜。

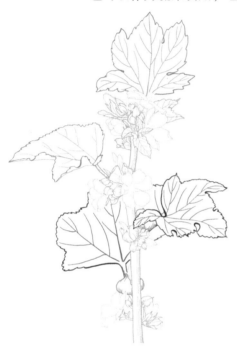

As long as we pay attention to the flower beds at the corner of the city, we can see a weed everywhere and it is a good herbal medicine around us. *Malva verticilata var. Crispa* L. is a biennial herb of the mallow family, people also call it Tuhuangqi, actually its herbal name is called Yekui. It is edible as vegetable and called winter Chinese mallow or amaranth.

冬葵在我国的分布很广，从南到北、从东到西到处都可以见到，它的茎、叶、根和种子都可以入药。其根味甘，性寒，无毒，具有清热、解毒、通淋的功效。作为蔬菜，冬葵在我国的河北、甘肃、江西、湖北、湖南等地有大面积的栽种。其叶片不仅是口感滑润的蔬菜，更是一味很好的草药，其味甘，性寒，具有清热、利湿、润肠、通乳的功效，可以用它来治疗肺热咳嗽、咽喉肿痛、热毒下痢、湿热黄疸、二便不通、乳汁不下、疮疖痈肿和丹毒。

Malva verticilata var. Crispa L. has a wide range of distribution in China, its stems, leaves, roots and seeds can be used as medicine, its root tastes sweet and non-toxic with cold property. It has the effects of clearing heat, detoxifying and treating stranguria. *Malva verticilata var. Crispa* L. is largely planted as a vegetable in Hebei, Gansu, Jiangxi, Hubei, Hunan and Southwest of China, its leaves are not only a vegetable with smooth taste, but also a good herbal medicine with sweet taste and cold property. It has the effects of clearing heat, removing dampness, moistening intestine and promoting lactation and it can be used to treat cough caused by lung heat, swollen sore throat, diarrhea caused by heat poison, jaundice due to damp-heat, anuria and constipation, breast milk stoppage, sore and furuncle abscess as well as erysipelas.

冬葵既可以煎汤，鲜品也可以捣汁内服，外用可以捣敷或者研末调敷，或煎水含漱。脾虚肠滑的患者禁用，孕妇也要慎用。

Malva verticilata var. Crispa L. can be decocted or its fresh leaves can be mashed into juice for taking internally, it can also be mashed or grinded into fine powder to apply on the skin for external use, or it can even be used as gargle after being decoted. While patients with spleen deficiency and slip of intestine are forbidden to use it, and pregnant women should take it with caution.

冬葵子，也叫葵子或者是葵菜子，就是冬葵的果实，其味甘，性寒，具有利水通淋、润肠通便和通乳的功效。可以用它来治疗淋证、水肿、大便不通，产妇乳汁不足。冬葵子入药一般煎汤内服，也可以入丸散，脾虚腹泻的患者和孕妇禁用。

Except its roots and leaves, the seeds of *Malva verticilata var. Crispa* L., are also commonly used in Chinese medicine. It is a common medicine which is stored in the general hospitals and pharmacies. The seeds of Melvacrispa L. are the fruit of Melvacrispa L. and is known as cluster mallow fruit or sunflower seed. It tastes sweet with cold property and has the effects of relieving stranguria, moistening intestine and relaxing bowel as well as promoting lactation. Therefore, its seeds can be used to treat gonorrhea, edema, constipation and galactostasis. It is generally taken orally as medicine after decoction, and it can also be grinded into powder to make pill, patients with diarrhea due to spleen deficiency and pregnant women are forbidden to use.

通过现代药理研究的不断发现，冬葵子是一味具有很好的临床运用价值和研究价值的中药。

Seeds of *Malva verticilata var. Crispa* L. Can be used as traditional Chinese medicine with good clinical application value and research value after continuous studies of modern pharmacological researches.

11. 红花月见草

Oenothera rosea L′Hér. ex Aiton.

红花月见草，又称粉花月见草，是月见草的一种。原产于美国得克萨斯州南部和墨西哥，如今逸散到江西、广西、贵州、云南等地。以其根或全草入药，味苦，性凉，具有解毒，化瘀，降压的功效，主治热毒疮肿，冠心病，高血压症。

Oenothera rosea L′Hér. ex Aiton. is native to South Texas and Mexico and now it is spreaded to Jiangxi, Guangxi, Guizhou, Yunnan. Using its roots or whole plant as medicine, it tastes bitter with cold property and has the effects of detoxifying, dispersing blood stasis and reducing blood pressure. It can be used to treat heat toxic sores, coronary heart disease and hypertension.

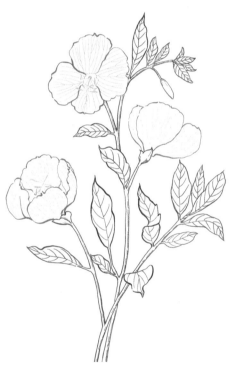

12. 灰藋（藜）　　*Chenopodium album* L.

　　灰藋在民间叫灰灰菜，它不仅是一种可口的野菜，还是一味很好的中药，入药部分为藜科藜属植物藜的全草。灰灰菜又叫灰条菜、灰苋菜，它的分布很广，除了西藏以外，全国大部分省区都能见到。在《中药大词典》和《中华本草》当中，灰灰菜的中药名叫灰藋。其味苦、甘，性平，具有祛风，清热，解毒，祛湿和杀虫的功效。灰藋治病既可以煎汤内服，也可以煎水外洗或者是捣烂外敷。

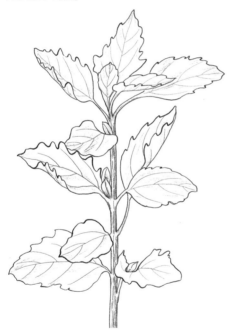

Chenopodium album L. is called Huihuicai, it is not only a delicious wild vegetable, but also a good herbal medicine, its whole herb of Chenopodiumalbum L. can be used as medicine. Huihuicai is also called Huitiaocai or Huixiancai, it is widely distributed and can be found in most provinces of China except the Tibet Autonomous region. Its medicinal name is called Huidiao in *the Dictionary of Chinese Materia Medica* and *Chinese Herbal Medicine*. It tastes bitter and sweet with mild property and has the effects of dispelling wind-evil, clearing heat, detoxifying, dispelling dampness and killing insects. *Chenopodium album* L. can be taken orally after being decoted, or wash externally after being boiled, or mashed and applied externally.

13. 金银花

Lonicera japonia Thunb.

自古以来，金银花因其药用价值而闻名，其清热解毒的功效被人们熟知，并在临床上普遍使用。中药金银花为忍冬科忍冬属植物忍冬的干燥花蕾或初开的花。几十年来，金银花的现代药理研究特别多，其抗炎解热、抗菌、抗病毒的研究已被临床和实验室证明。

Lonicera japoniaflos is well known for its medicinal value and its heat-clearing and detoxification effect and widely used in clinical practice. The medicinal part of the *Lonicera japoniaflos* that used as medicine are its dry buds or the first blossoms of *Lonicera japonica* Thunb. There were numerous modern pharmacological researches on *Lonicera japoniaflos* in recent decades, its anti-inflammatory, antipyretic, antibacterial and antiviral studies have been proved clinically and experimentally.

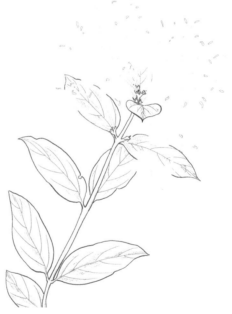

其实，金银花的功效还有很多：其水提取物表现出良好的体外抗氧化作用，还有研究显示，金银花对呼吸系统具有抗癌和保护作用。此外，金银花还有明显的保肝、降血糖、神经保护，以及增强免疫功能等多方面的作用，小小一朵金银花，还需要我们进一步去研究和发掘它的临床效用。

In fact, *Lonicera japoniaflos* has many other effects. Firstly, its water extract showed excellent antioxidant activity effect in vitro and other studies showed that *Lonicera japoniaflos* has anti-cancer and protective effects on the respiratory system. In addition, *Lonicera japoniaflos* also has obvious liver protection, blood sugar level regulating, neuro protection and immune function enhancing. Although *Lonicera japoniaflos* is a tiny and small flower, it is worthy our further studying and exploring on its clinical effectiveness.

14. 马鞭草

Verbena officinalis L.

马鞭草可能很少有人不知道，它也是一味大家随处可见的中药。马鞭草有很多名字：马鞭梢、马鞭、铁马鞭、小铁马鞭，它在我国的分布非常广泛，在中南、西南和西北地区以及华东的江浙、华南一带都有分布。只要你留意山坡、路边、沟边和草地，到处都有马鞭草的身影。

Only a few people may familiar with *Verbena officinalis* L., it is a common Chinese herbal medicine and can be found everywhere. It is also called Mabianshao, Mabian, Tiemabian or Xiaotiemabian, it is widely distributed in Central and South China, Southwest and Northwest China, Jiangsu and Zhejiang provinces as well as South China, and it can be found everywhere on hillsides, roadsides, ditches and meadows.

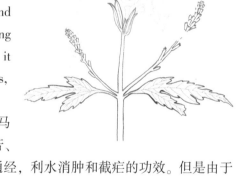

马鞭草的入药部位为马鞭草科马鞭草属植物马鞭草的全草，其味苦、辛，性微寒，具有清热解毒，活血通经，利水消肿和截疟的功效。但是由于马鞭草有活血通经的作用，孕妇是不能使用的。

The whole plant of the genus and family *Verbena officinalis* L. can be used as herbal medicine, it tastes bitter and pungent with minor cold property, and it has the effects of clearing heat and detoxifying, promoting blood circulation and regulating meridian, alleviating edema and stopping malaria. While pregnant woman is forbidden to use it due to its blood circulation function.

马鞭草是一种低毒有效，而且资源非常丰富的草药，值得我们高度关注。

Verbenaofficinalis L. is rich in resources and effective herbal medicine with low toxicity, which deserves our high attention.

15. 苦刺（白刺花）

Sophora davidii kom. ex Pavol

白刺花，又名苦刺、苦刺花、狼牙刺，是云南人最喜爱的山珍，从小长辈就告诉我们苦刺花味道虽苦，但是它是清火的。这种豆科苦参属植物的根、叶、花以及它的果实，都是我们的中药，其味苦，性寒。它的根具有清热解毒、利湿消肿和凉血止血的功效。苦刺花的果实具有理气消积的功效，苦刺花的花朵既可以做茶饮，也可以做菜吃，它具有清凉解暑的功效。

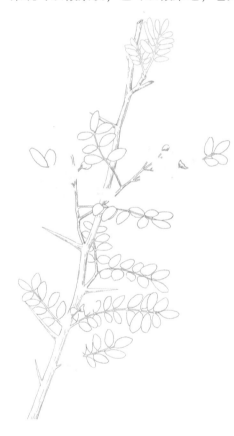

Sophora davidii kom. ex Pavol is the favorite mountain treasure of Yunnan people. The elders told us that it tastes bitter, but it can clear the heat in our body. It is called Kuci or Langyaci and its roots, leaves, flowers as well as fruits can be used as medicine, they taste bitter with cold property. Its roots have the effects of clearing heat and detoxifying, alleviating edema, cooling blood and stopping bleeding, its fruits have the effects of regulating Qi and eliminating stagnation, and its flowers can be used to make tea drink or cook as dishes for relieving summer-heat.

现代药理研究发现，苦刺花的根和叶含有槐果碱，槐果碱具有抗癌、抗过敏和平喘的作用。

Modern pharmacological studies showed that the roots and leaves of *Sophora davidii* kom. ex Pavol contain sophocarpine that has the effects of anti-cancer, anti-allergy and anti-asthmatics.

16. 泽漆

Euphorbia helioscopia L.

泽漆有很多名字：五朵云、猫眼草、五凤草、登台草。这种大戟科草本植物的全草，都可以入药，其味辛、苦，微寒，有毒，具有利水消肿、化痰止咳、散结和杀虫的功效。作为常用中药，泽漆在临床上常被用于治疗腹水、水肿、肺结核，也可以治疗淋巴结结核、痰多、咳喘，各种皮肤病和肿瘤。

Wuduoyun, Maoyancao, Wufengcao and Dengtaicao are the alias of *Euphorbia helioscopia* L., which belongs to euphorbia family and its whole plant can be used as medicine. It is poisonous and tastes pungent and bitter with minor cold, it has the effects of alleviating edema, resolving phlegm and relieving cough, eliminating stasis and killing insects. As a commonly used Chinese medicine, it is often used clinically to treat ascites, edema, pulmonary tuberculosis, lymph node tuberculosis, excessive phlegm, cough and asthma, as well as various skin diseases and tumors.

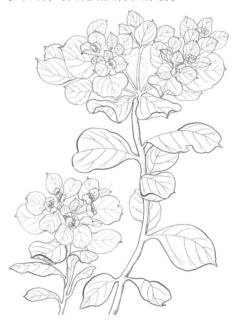

但是作为大戟科植物，它对人体是有一定毒性的，它的乳状汁液对皮肤、黏膜有很强的刺激性，可使皮肤发炎甚至溃烂。如果食用其鲜草或者白色乳汁，可以使口腔、食管、胃黏膜发生炎症糜烂，而出现灼痛、恶心、呕吐、腹痛、腹泻、水样便，严重者还会出现脱水甚至酸中毒。

However, as an aeuphorbiaceae plant, it is toxic to human and its milky juice has a strong irritation to the skin and mucosa, which may make the skin inflamed or even ulcerated. If we take its fresh grass or white milk, it will cause inflammation and erosion of the oral cavity, esophagus and stomach mucosa, and there will be burning pain, nausea, vomiting, abdominal pain, diarrhea, watery stool, and even dehydration or acidosis for severe cases.

作为一味有毒中药，泽漆不可过量使用，气血虚弱者也不要使用。

As a toxic herbal medicine, it cannot be overused and people who suffers from Qi deficiency and blood weakness are forbidden to use it.

17. 黄锁梅（栽秧藨）

Rubus ellipticus var. *obcordatus*（Franch.）Focke

这种在云南路边常见的小果子，是很多孩子的最爱，虽然采摘它的果实时，往往会被它的倒钩刺扎伤，但是在那种夏季炎热环境下，小果子酸甜凉爽的诱惑，是小小倒钩刺无法阻挡的。黄锁梅是蔷薇科悬钩子属的灌木，学名叫栽秧藨，别名黄锁梅、黄泡，它的根叶和果实是我们身边的草药，其中药名叫黄锁梅，属于中药当中的收涩药，其功效和性能相当于中药覆盆子。

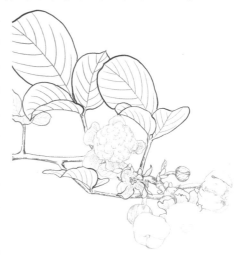

The small fruit commonly seen on the roadsides in Yunnan was the favorite fruit of many children when they were young, although they might be stabbed by its barb thorns when picking it, its sour and sweet tastes and the feeling of refreshing after taking them in hot summer, the small barb thorns were unable to hold back their temptation. *Rubus ellipticus* var. *obcordatus*（Franch.）Focke is the shrub of the genus Myrtaceae, it is also called Huangsuomei or Huangpao. Its roots, leaves and fruits are herbs around us, and its medicinal name is called Huangsuomei, which belongs to the astringent medicine in Chinese medicine, and its efficacy and property are equivalent to raspberry.

春夏季将其采摘洗净，晒干以后就可以入药，除了果实以外，黄锁梅的叶和根也是很好的草药，每逢秋季将其采挖，洗净切片，晒干以后就可以入药。其味酸涩，性温，具有消肿止痛、收涩止泻的功效。

Collect its fruits in spring and summer, it can be used as medicine after being washed thoroughly and dried in the sun. Except for its fruits, the leaves and roots of the Huangsuomei are also very good herbs, dig and collect its roots every autumn, then wash and slice them into pieces, they can be used as medicine after being dried in the sun. They taste sour and astringent with warm property and they can relieve swelling and pain, induce astringency and relieve diarrhea.

18. 鼠曲草

Pseadog naphalium affine（D. Don）Anderb.

鼠曲草在我国的分布非常广泛，所有南方省区和大部分北方地区都有分布，在云南更是到处可见。它不仅是云南人常摘回家做美食的原料，也是我们身边的草药，这种菊科一年生草本植物的全草都是其入药部位，其味甘、微酸，性平，归肺经，具有化痰止咳，祛风除湿，解毒的功效，主治咳喘痰多，风湿痹痛、泄泻、水肿、蚕豆病、赤白带下、痈肿疔疮、阴囊湿痒、荨麻疹、高血压。

Pseadog naphalium affine (D. Don) Anderb. is widely distributed in southern provinces and most of northern regions, and it can be found everywhere in Yunnan. It is not only the delicious tish for Yunnan people, but also a common herb around us. The whole plant of this annual herb of Compositae family can be used as medicine, it tastes sweet and slightly acidic with mild property, and belongs to lung meridian. It has the effects of eliminating phlegm and relieving cough, dispelling wind evil and removing dampness, detoxifying, and it can be used to treat cough and asthma with excessive phlegm, rheumatism and arthralgia, diarrhea, edema, favism, leukorrhea with reddish discharge, abscess and pustule, wet itch of scrotum, urticaria and hypertension.

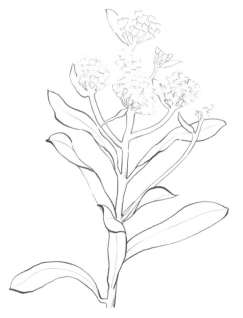

19. 覆盆子

Rubus idaeus L.

　　覆盆子为蔷薇科悬钩子属植物华东覆盆子的未成熟果实。覆盆子和黄锁梅同科同属，功效和主治也非常相似。关于覆盆子名称的由来有很多说法，其中有一个传说，就是覆盆子的名称与中国古代名医葛洪有关。传说一次偶然的机会，葛洪在山上采摘了这种红果食用，意想不到的是竟然治愈了他多年的夜尿症。服用了这种果子后，有夜尿症的人可以在晚上将夜尿盆翻过来放置，不需要使用夜尿盆了。所以，葛洪就把这种小野果取名覆盆子。

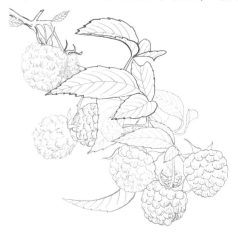

　　Rubus idaeus L. is the unripe fruit of the genus Rubus of the rose family, and it has the same family and genus as well as the same efficacy and indications with Duranta repens cv. Gold leaves. There are many legends about the origin of the name of the *Rubus idaeus* L. and one of the legends is related to a famous ancient Chinese doctor Ge Hong, he picked this red fruit and ate it by chance, his old trouble of nocturia was cured unexpectedly after taking it, so people suffer from nocturia can turn over the nocturia basin and do not need to use it anymore. Therefore, Ge Hong named this small wild fruit Fupenzi.

　　覆盆子的入药部位就是它的果实，每当初夏之际，将其果实洗净、晒干就可以入药了。其味甘、酸，性温，具有益肾固精、养肝明目的功效，主治肾气不足、下元虚冷而致遗精、滑精、遗尿、尿频、阳痿、不孕，以及肝肾不足，两目昏花，视物不清等。

　　The medicinal part of *Rubus idaeus* L. is its fruits, they can be used as medicine after being washed and dried in the sun during early summer. It tastes sweet and sour with mild property and it has the effects of tonifying kidney and reinforcing essence, nourishing liver and brightening eyes. It can be used to treat deficiency of kidney Qi, nocturnal emission, night essonce, enuresis, frequent urination, impotence and infertility due to the deficiency of vital Qi, deficiency of liver and kidney, as well as dimness with blurred vision.

20. 天南星

Arisaema erubescens（Wall.）schott

"南星一把伞，半夏三匹叶"，这是流传于云南民间最朴素易记的认药、识药口诀。这里所说的"南星"实际上是"一把伞南星"，它就是我们说的中药"天南星"的首选植物来源。

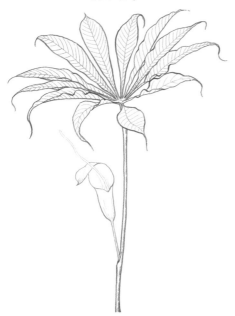

Arisaema erubescens（Wall.）schott looks like an umbrella and Pinellia ternata has three pieces of leaves, this is a simple and easy herb recognition formula widely spread among Yunnan people to distinguish Araceae from Pinellia ternate. *Arisaema erubescens*（Wall.）Schott is the preferred plant source for the traditional Chinese medicine Tiannanxing.

一把伞南星是茎块入药，由于它有很大的毒性，所以我们一般是不生用的，生用不当非常容易中毒，从而出现口腔黏膜的溃烂，唇、舌、咽喉麻木肿胀甚至出现锁喉。一把伞南星中毒还可以出现：大量流涎、言语不清、发热头昏、心慌、四肢麻木，严重的还可能出现昏迷，惊厥，窒息和呼吸停止。所以在这里提醒大家，一定要在医生的指导下使用一把伞南星。

The stems of Arisaema erubescens can be used as medicine, while it cannot be used raw due to its strong toxicity. It may cause the ulceration of the oral mucosa, numbness and swelling of the lip, tongue and throat or even throat choke if it is used raw improperly. In addition, symptoms such as excessive salivation, slurred speech, fever, dizziness, panic, numbness of limbs, and even coma, convulsions, suffocation and respiratory arrest may also appear. Therefore, it is should be used carefully under the guidance of doctor.

中医临床上通常将它炮制以后和其他药物配伍使用，用量一般是3—9克，煎汤服用。南星具有燥湿化痰、祛风止痉、散结消肿的作用，常用于顽痰咳嗽、风痰眩晕、中风、口眼㖞斜、半身不遂、癫痫、惊风、破伤风等。现代研究发现南星具有明显的抗肿瘤的作用，可以用于颅内肿瘤、鼻咽癌、肺癌等；南星还具有祛痰镇静、抗惊厥、抗心律失常、抗氧化等多种药理作用。由于它属于毒麻药物，性温，燥烈，所以孕妇、阴虚内热或者是实热证、血虚动风的患者，是不能使用的。

Arisaema erubescens is usually used with other pharmaceutical compounds after being processed in clinical practice, the dosage is generally 3—9 grams, take it orally after being decocted, it has the effects of drying dampness and resolving phlegm, expelling wind and relieving spasm, dispersing stasis and reducing swelling. It is commonly used to treat stubborn sputum cough, wind sputum dizziness, stroke, facial paralysis, hemiplegia, epilepsy, convulsions and tetanus. Modern studies have found that Arisaema erubescens has obvious anti-tumor effect and can be used for intracranial tumors, nasopharyngeal and lung cancer, as well as pharmacological effects of expectorant sedation, anti-convulsion, anti-arrhythmia and anti-oxidation. Arisaema erubescens is a kind of narcotic herb with warm property, therefore, pregnant women and patients suffer from internal heat due to Yin deficiency, solid heat syndrome, blood deficiency are forbidden to use.

21. 余甘子

Phyllanthusemblica L.

余甘子在云南山间经常可见，当地人食用它的果实来解暑解渴。余甘子味甘、酸涩，性凉，具有清热凉血、健胃消食、生津止渴、消暑止咳的功效。临床上可用余甘子 3—9 克煎汤内服，用于治疗消化不良、腹胀、咳嗽、咳吐黄痰、口干口渴、咽喉肿痛、感冒发热以及因血热引起的鼻衄、咳血等。

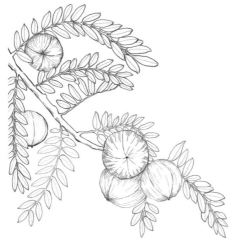

Phyllanthusemblica L. is often seen in the mountains of Yunnan province, local people consume its fruits to quench their thirst and heat. It tastes sweet, sour and astringent with cold property and it has the effects of clearing heat and cooling blood, strengthening stomach and promoting digestion, promoting the secretion of saliva to quench thirst, refreshing summer heat and relieving cough. Decoct 3—9 grams of Phyllanthi Frutns. and take it orally to treat dyspepsia, abdominal distension, cough, cough with spit yellow phlegm, dry mouth and thirst, swollen and sore throat, cold and fever, as well as epistaxis and hemoptysis caused by blood heat.

除此之外，余甘子的根、树皮、叶也可以入药，它的根常用来消食、利水消肿、化痰杀虫，可以用来治疗高血压、腹泻、瘰疬也就是淋巴结肿大。余甘子的叶常被用来去湿利尿，常用于治疗水肿、皮肤湿疹，临床上根的用量在 30 克以内，叶的用量在 15 克以内，煎汤内服，也可以将它捣烂外敷，或者是煮水外洗。需要提醒大家的是，余甘子性凉而且其根有毒，脾胃虚寒的人一定要慎重使用。

In addition, its roots, barks and leaves can also be used as medicine. Its roots are commonly used to promote food digestion, alleviate edema by inducing diuresis, eliminate phlegm and kill insects, as well as cure hypertension, diarrhea and scrofula. And its leaves are often used to remove dampness and promote diuresis, treat edema and skin tinea and eczema. Clinically, the amount of root used in medicine is less than 30 grams, and the amount of leaf is no more than 15 grams, decocting and taking it orally, or it can also be mashed for external application, or boiled its water for external washing. People with spleen and stomach deficiency should use it with caution due to its cold property and its roots are poisonous.

现代研究发现余甘子富含维生素 C，所以它具有抗氧化和延缓衰老的作用，它富含的单磷酸既可以吸收紫外线，又能够分解多余的黑色素，促进细胞的新陈代谢和收缩毛孔，所以余甘子有美肤的作用。由于余甘子富含各种矿物元素，如钙、铁、磷、钾、硒，所以它还具有抗心血管疾病和防癌的作用。余甘子还有调节胃肠菌群，抑制血糖升高，降低胆固醇等作用。

Modern research has found that *Phyllanthusemblica* L. is rich in vitamin C, so it has antioxidant and anti-aging effects, its rich monophoric acid can absorb ultraviolet rays, but can also decompose excess melanin, promote cell metabolism and shrink pores, so *Phyllanthusemblica* L. also has the effect of skin care. Because *Phyllanthusemblica* L. is abundant with various mineral elements, such as calcium, iron, phosphorus, potassium, and selenium, so it also has anti-cardiovascular disease and anti-cancer effects as well as the functions of regulating gastrointestinal flora, inhibiting the rise of blood sugar and reducing cholesterol.

很多云南人到了夏天，会用晒干的余甘子来泡茶饮用。余甘子不仅是一种很好的中药，它又是一种营养十分丰富的果实，由于其性寒凉，所以脾胃虚寒和大便稀薄的朋友不能过量服用，孕妇也要慎重服用。云南很多老百姓习惯用余甘子来泡酒饮，但是过量服用余甘子酒，会有维生素 C 中毒的可能，所以虽然余甘子是好东西，但是也不可多食。

Yunnan people often use the dried *Phyllanthusemblica* L. to make tea drinking in summer. *Phyllanthusemblica* L. is indeed a good Chinese medicine, and it is also a fruit with rich nutrition, while people who suffer from spleen and stomach deficiency with loose stool cannot take it excessively, and pregnant women should take it with caution. Yunnan people are used to infuse it in liquor, but taking it excessively may cause vitamin C poisoning, therefore, although *Phyllanthusemblica* L. is a good fruit, it cannot be taken too much.

22. 苏木

Biancaea sappan（L.）Tod.

中药饮片苏木为豆科云实属植物苏木的干燥心材，是传统的中药。原植物苏木豆科的常绿乔本植物，在云南的滇中和滇南都有分布，它的干燥心材，也就是将其枝干的外皮和边材除去，干燥加工后的部分，就是其入药部位。作为中药，苏木味甘、咸，性平，具有行血、破瘀、消肿、止痛的功效，在临床上一般用3—12克煎汤内服，也可以研末服用或者是研末外撒患处。临床上常用于治疗妇女的血滞经闭、痛经、产后瘀阻导致的胸腹疼痛、瘀血导致的胸腹刺痛、外伤肿痛、跌打损伤、痢疾等病症。

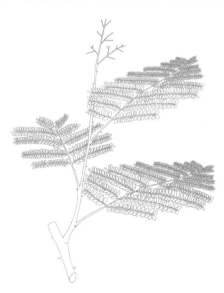

Sappan Lignum is the dried heartwood of Caesalpinia decapetala (Roth) Alston and a traditional herbal medicine. The evergreen legume plant is distributed in central and southern Yunnan and its dried heartwood is used as medicinal part by removing the outer skin and sapwood of its branches after beign dried and processed. It tastes sweet and salty with mild property, it has the effects of promoting blood circulation, eliminating blood stasis, reducing swelling and relieving pain. Decoct 3—12 grams and take it orally in clinical practice or spread it on the wound after being grinded. It can also be used to treat amenorrhea due to blood stagnation, dysmenorrhea, chest and abdominal pain caused by postpartum stasis, tingling pain in the chest and abdomen due to congestion, traumatic swelling pain, traumatic injury and dysentery.

现代药理研究发现，苏木还具有抗肿瘤的作用以及免疫抑制的作用，同时苏木还具有抗菌、消炎、抗氧化、降血糖的作用。在云南很多少数民族都把苏木用作补益强壮的药物来使用，认为苏木具有强身健体、延缓衰老的作用，所以在傣族地区，人们常用苏木来当茶饮。在云南很多少数民族都把苏木用于治疗全身乏力、性欲冷淡、阳痿、遗精、早泄以及慢性肠炎、痢疾、高血压、心慌、心悸、贫血等病症。

Modern pharmacological research found that Sappan Lignum also has the effects of antitumor, immuno suppression, antibacterial, anti-inflammatory, antioxidant and regulating blood sugar level. Many ethnic minorities in Yunnan often use it as a tonic medicine and believe that it has the effects of strengthening the body and delaying senility, so Dai people often drink it as tea. Furthermore, many ethnic minorities in Yunnan also use it to treat malaise, apathy, impotence, emission, premature ejaculation, chronic enteritis, dysentery, hypertension, palpitation and anemia.

苏木作为传统中药，它具有活血化瘀、消肿止痛的功效，所以临床上常用它来治疗跌打损伤、闭经以及心腹疼痛等病症。随着现代研究的不断深入，其临床运用领域也在不断地拓展，尤其在抗菌、消炎、抗肿瘤、降血糖、抗氧化等多方面，对苏木都有了新的认识。

As a traditional Chinese medicine, Sappan Lignum has the effects of promoting blood circulation, removing blood stasis, reducing swelling and relieving pain, so it is widely used to treat traumatic injuries, amenorrhea and abdominal pain Clinically. With the deepening of modern research, its clinical applications are also incessantly expanded, especially in antibacterial, anti-inflammatory, anti-tumor, regulating blood sugar level and antioxidant.

23. 大叶钩藤 *Uncaria macrophylla* Wall. in Roxb

大叶钩藤主要分布在我国广西、广东、云南、海南等热带亚热带地区。这种茜草科钩藤属大藤本植物在云南也有人把它当作钩藤使用，同时它还是一味著名的傣药。大叶钩藤的入药部位就是带钩的茎枝。它味苦、微涩，性凉，具有清火解毒、消肿止痛、祛风及通气血的功效。临床上常用它来治疗风湿热痹，也就是肢体关节红肿、热痛、屈伸不利，也可以用它来治疗风寒湿痹，也就是肢体关节酸痛、冷痛、屈伸不利，还可以用来治疗头部胀痛。一般用15克以内的剂量煎汤内服，但不可久煎。

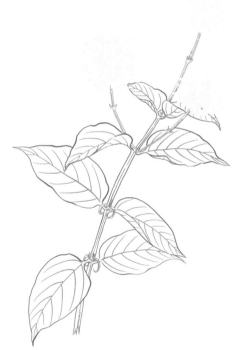

Uncaria macrophylla Wall. is mainly distributed in Guangxi, Guangdong, Yunnan, Hainan and other tropical and subtropical regions. The rubiaceae, unguia genus of large vine plant is also used as Uncariae Pamulus Cum Uncis in Yunnan and it is also one of the famous Dai herbal medicines. Its stirps with hook are used as medicine and they taste bitter and minor astringent with cold property. It has the effects of clearing heat and detoxifying, relieving swelling and pain, dispelling wind pathogen and regulating Qi and blood. It is commonly used to treat rheumatic fever arthralgia clinically, that is, red and swollen of limb joints heat pain, unfavorable flexion and extension, and it can also be used to treat limb joint pain, cold pain, unfavorable flexion and extension as well as treat head swelling and pain. Generally, decoct 15 grams or less of Uncaria macrophylla Wall. and take it internally, but it can not be decoted for too long.

现代研究发现，大叶钩藤具有降血压和镇静安神的作用，同时对热证抽搐有预防作用。在云南西双版纳，还有一种毛钩藤，它的果实长相奇特，有点像高倍镜下冠状病毒的模样。毛钩藤和大叶钩藤是同科、同属、同种的植物，都属于钩藤的正品，不同之处就是它们的长相。大叶钩藤因其叶大而得名，它的叶子的长度可以达到十五六厘米，宽可以达到12厘米左右，而且正面的叶脉凹陷明显。而毛钩藤的叶最长也不过12厘米，宽也不超过五六厘米，叶面、叶背和叶柄都有毛。

Modern studies have found that *Uncaria macrophylla* Wall. has the effects of lowering blood pressure, tranquilizing and allaying, and it also has the preventive effect on heat syndrome convulsions. There is another Uncaria hirsuta in Xishuangbanna with peculiar fruits resembling the coronavirus under magnification. It belongs to the same family, genus and species of *Uncaria macrophylla* Wall. and the difference between them is their appearances, *Uncaria macrophylla* Wall. is named after the size of its leaves, its leaves can be 15—16cm in length and about 12cm in width with obvious sunken veins on the positive side, while the leaves of Uncaria hirsute is less than 12cm in length and less than 5—6cm in width with fur on the right side, the reverse side and stipe.

毛钩藤和大叶钩藤，它们的生长环境也非常相似，主要生长于热带、亚热带地区，在中国主要分布于广东、广西、海南、云南，由于毛钩藤比大叶钩藤耐寒，所以它在华东的江浙、华中、华南、西南等地也有分布。

In addition, *Uncaria macrophylla* Wall. and *Uncaria hirsute* Havil. grow in the similar environment, they mainly grow in tropical and subtropical areas and are mainly distributed in Guangdong, Guangxi, Hainan and Yunnan in China. Uncaria hirsute is also distributed in east China of Jiangsu and Zhejiang, central China, south China and Southwest China etc., due to its cold tolerance than Uncaria macrophylla Wall.

24. 紫苏

Perilla frutescens（L.）Britt.

中药饮片紫苏为唇形科紫苏属植物紫苏的茎、叶。其叶称为紫苏叶，其茎称为紫苏梗。紫苏原产于中国，在中国已有2000多年种植历史，分布范围广，中国各地均有栽培。味辛，性温，归肺、脾经，具有解表散寒、行气宽中、安胎、解鱼蟹毒的功效，主治风寒感冒，脾胃气滞、胸闷呕吐，胎气上逆、胎动不安、七情郁结、痰凝气滞之梅核气证，进食鱼蟹中毒而致腹痛吐泻等。

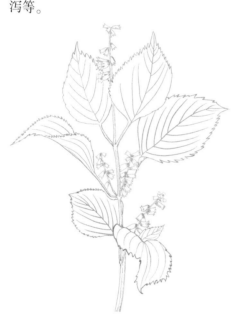

Chinese Medicine Perilla is the stems and leaves of the genus Perilla of the labiaceae family, its leaves are called Perilla leaves and the stems are called Perilla stems. *Perilla frutescens* （L.）Britt. is native to China and it has been cultivated in China for more than 2000 years. It is widely distributed and cultivated all over China. It tastes pungent with mild property and belongs to lung, spleen meridian, and it has the effects of dispelling surface cold, regulating Qi andexpanding channels, preventing miscarriage, detoxifying fish and crab poison, it is commonly used to treat wind-cold, Qi stagnation in the spleen and stomach, chest tightness and vomiting, reversed fetal air, fetal irritability, seven emotions depression, globus hystericus syndrome caused by phlegm congealing and Qi stagnation, abdominal pain, vomiting and diarrhea due to fish and crabs poisoning.

25. 铜锤玉带草

Lobelia nummularia Lam.

铜锤玉带草是一味记载于《云南民族药大词典》中的草药，也是云南很多少数民族都喜欢使用的一味草药。雨季的滇南遍地可见这种带紫色小果的草药，这种桔梗科多年生草本植物，不仅在云南有分布，在湖北、湖南两省，以及华东、华南西南各省也有分布。

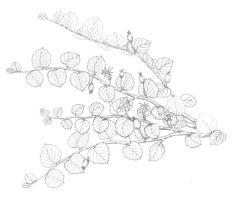

Tongchuiyudaicao. is one of the herbs that recorded in the *Dictionary of Yunnan Ethnic Medicine*, it is also a favourite herb for ethnic minorities in Yunnan. This herb with small purple fruits can be found all over southern Yunnan during the rainy season. It is the perennial herb of platycodon family, is also distributed in in east China of Jiangsu and Zhejiang, as well as, Hubei, Hunan, south China and southwest China.

在云南不同民族有不同的叫法，汉族叫它小铜锤扣子草，而白族则叫它地钮子、地茄子，彝族叫它地萍，佤族又叫它地石榴。

Lobelia nummularia Lam. has different names among different ethnic groups in Yunnan, such as the Han people call it Xiaotongchuikouzicao, Bai people call it Niuzi, Diqiezi, Yi people call it the Diping, and Wa people call it Dishiliu.

各民族在使用它入药的时候基本是一样的，它全草入药，其味辛、苦，性平，具有清热解毒、祛风除湿、活血散瘀的功效，将其煎汤内服或者是捣烂外敷，可以用来治疗咳嗽、腋下淋巴结肿大、子宫脱垂、风湿疼痛、眼结膜炎、小儿惊风等病症。也有民族医生将它用于治疗月经不调、男子遗精、目赤肿痛、跌打损伤、外伤出血、乳腺炎以及各种无名肿毒。

It is basically the same in the use of medicine by all ethnic groups and its whole plant can be used as herbal medicine, and it tastes pungent and bitter with mild property. It has the effects of clearing heat and removing toxicity, dispelling wind and removing dampness, promoting blood circulation and dispersing stasis. And it can be used to treat cough, underarm lymphadenectasis, metroptosis, rheumatic pain, eye conjunctivitis and febrile convulsion by taking its decocted soup internally or applying its mash for external use. It is also used in the treatment of menstrual disorders, spermatospermia, red swollen eyes, trauma injuries, traumatic bleeding, mastitis and variousnameless pyogenic infections.

26. 梁王茶

Metapanax delavayi（Franch.）J. Wen & Frodin

梁王茶是一种生长于云、贵、川西南三省的五加科的灌木植物。据说梁王茶的得名，是来源于元朝云南的蒙古梁王以及昆明周边的梁王山的一段故事。传说梁王的士兵们，常把长在梁王山上的一种绿色植物拿来当茶喝，饮用后都觉神清气爽，于是就把这种植物叫作梁王茶。云南当地老百姓也把梁王茶拿来当野菜吃。梁王茶也是一味草药，其味甘、苦，性凉，具有清热解毒、活血舒筋的功效，可以用它来治疗咽喉肿痛、目赤肿痛、消化不良、月经不调、风湿腰腿疼痛、跌打损伤以及骨折。

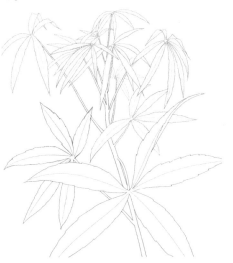

Metapanax delavayi(Franch.) J. Wen & Frodin is a kind of shrub plant of Acanthaceae, which grows in Yunnan, Guizhou and Sichuan provinces. It is said that the name of Liangwangcha comes from a story about the Mongolian King Liang in Yunnan in the Yuan Dynasty and the Liangwang Mountain near Kunming, the soldiers of King Liang often drank a kind of green plant as tea growing on the mountain, and they all felt refreshed after drinking it, so they called this plant Liangwangcha. Local people in Yunnan also take Liangwangcha as a wild vegetable. It is also an herb and tastes sweet and bitter with cold property; it has the effects of clearing heat and detoxifying, activating blood and relaxing tendons and it can be used to treat sore throat, red swollen eyes, dyspepsia, irregular menstruation, rheumatism, rheumatic waist and leg pain, injuries and fractures.

现代药理研究发现，梁王茶还有很多的药理活性，它所含的五环三萜物质，具有很好的抗癌、抗肿瘤、免疫调节、消炎镇痛、抗菌、抗病毒，以及防止心脑血管疾病的作用。梁王茶当中还含有一定比例的可溶性多糖，其多糖成分具有显著的消炎、抗衰老以及免疫双向调节的作用。有学者研究发现，梁王茶当中的可溶性多糖的提取率非常高，比同科植物刺五加高出 10 倍以上，有很好的开发运用价值。此外，梁王茶的嫩茎和嫩叶都是可口的蔬菜，根茎也是一味中药，是名副其实的药食同源。

Modern pharmacological studies have found that Liangwangcha has many pharmacological activities, and the pentacyclic triterpenoids contained in it have the effects of anti-cancer, anti-tumor, immune regulation, anti-inflammatory and analgesic, antibacterial, antiviral and prevention of cardiovascular and cerebrovascular diseases. There is also a certain proportion of soluble polysaccharide contained in it, and its polysaccharide components have significant anti-inflammatory, anti-aging and bidirectional immune regulation. Some scholars have found that the extraction rate of soluble polysaccharide in Liangwangcha is very high, which is more than 10 times higher than that of Acanthopanax in the same family, and it owns the value for future development and application. In addition, its tender stems and leaves are tasty vegetable and its roots are also a traditional Chinese medicine, which is the real representative of the homology of medicine and food.

27. 玉竹

Polygonatum odoratum(Mill.)Druce

玉竹是百合科多年生草本植物的根茎，是一味常用的中药。玉竹味甘，性微寒，具有养阴润燥、生津止渴的功效，临床上常用它来治疗肺胃阴伤、燥热咳嗽，以及咽喉干燥和内热消渴。现代药理研究发现，玉竹具有稳定血压的作用，同时它还能够强心和抗心肌缺血、调节血糖、治疗冠状动脉粥样硬化。玉竹还具有提高机体免疫力、调节造血的功效。

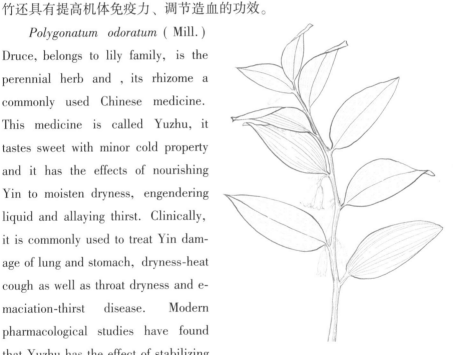

Polygonatum odoratum (Mill.) Druce, belongs to lily family, is the perennial herb and , its rhizome a commonly used Chinese medicine. This medicine is called Yuzhu, it tastes sweet with minor cold property and it has the effects of nourishing Yin to moisten dryness, engendering liquid and allaying thirst. Clinically, it is commonly used to treat Yin damage of lung and stomach, dryness-heat cough as well as throat dryness and e-maciation-thirst disease. Modern pharmacological studies have found that Yuzhu has the effect of stabilizing blood pressure, and it can also strengthen the heart and anti-myocardial ischemi-a, regulate blood sugar and treat coronary atherosclerosis. In addition, it can also enhance the body immunity and regulate hematopoiesis.

现代研究证明玉竹有明显的降血糖的作用，让实验家兔口服玉竹浸膏，会使家兔出现血糖先升后降的情况。玉竹的甲醇提取物水溶部分能够明显降低实验小鼠的血糖，并显示有改善耐糖功能的倾向。另外玉竹还具有扩张血管的作用，研究证明玉竹注射液对蟾蜍下肢血管有明显的扩张作用。还有很多实验证明，玉竹对血压有调节作用，同时对心肌也有一定的保护作用。

Modern studies have proved that Yuzhu has obvious hypoglycemic effect. The blood glucose of experimental rabbits may rise first and then fall after taking Yuzhu extract orally. The water-soluble part of methanol extract can significantly reduce the blood sugar of experimental mice and show a tendency to improve glucose tolerance. Furthermore, Yuzhu also has the effect of vasodilation, and it has been proved that Yuzhu injection has the obvious effect of vasodilation on the lower limbs of toad. There are also many experiments that have proved that Yuzhu can regulate blood pressure, and it also has a certain protective effect on myocardium.

玉竹不仅是一味滋阴润肺、养阴生津的中药，而且对心血管系统、血糖、血脂、免疫系统也有一定的作用，现代研究大大拓宽了中医临床使用玉竹的范围和适应证。

Yuzhu is not only a traditional Chinese medicine for tonifying Yin and moistening lung, nourishing Yin and engendering fluid, but also has certain effects on cardiovascular system, blood glucose and lipids, and immune system. Modern researches have greatly expanded the scope and applications of clinical use of Yuzhu in traditional Chinese medicine.

28. 咳地佬(诃子) *Terminalia chebula* Retz

咳地佬又称诃子、随风子，为使君子科榄仁树属植物诃子的成熟果实。在中国分布于云南西部和西南部，广东、广西也有栽培。在滇西经常见到有人把这种果实拿来做菜吃，当地人把它叫作咳地佬，滇西百姓除了拿咳地佬泡酒和炖肉吃以外，放些辣椒和佐料腌制做果脯也是常见的。

Kedilao is also called Hezi or Suifengzi, it is the mature fruits of combretaceae tropical almond plant of *Terminalia chebula* Retz. It is distributed in western and southwestern Yunnan, and cultivated in Guangdong and Guangxi. In western Yunnan, people often take this kind of fruits as their dishes and call it Kedilao, they often soak it in liquor for drinking or stew it with meat to eat, or they may make preserved fruit by adding some chili and seasoning.

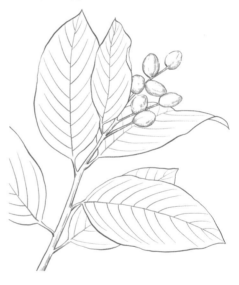

作为中药，诃子味苦、酸、涩，性平，归肺、大肠经，具有涩肠止泻，敛肺止咳，利咽开音的功效，主治久泻久痢、便血脱肛、肺虚喘咳、久咳不止、咽痛音哑。

As an herbal medicine, it tastes bitter, sour and astringent with mild property, it attributes to lung and large intestine meridian. It has the effects of astringing intestine to stop diarrhea, moistening lung to stop cough and relieving sore throat. It is mainly used to treat chronic diarrhea and dysentery, hematochezia and rectocele, panting cough due to lung deficiency, chronic cough and sore throat with hoarseness.

29. 天胡荽　　　*Hydrocotyle sibthorpioides* Lam.

天胡荽是一种在草地、湿地、沟边经常可以见到的小草，也是我们身边的一种草药。云南人也叫它破铜钱、破现、线草、满天星、肺风草、鸡肠菜。天胡荽入药部分为伞形科植物天胡荽的全草。在我国的长江以南的各省区都有分布，只要把这种草搓揉以后，就会散发出一种特殊的味道。这种伞形科匍匐生的草本植物，全草皆可入药。其味辛、微苦，性凉，具有清热利湿、解毒消肿的功效，主治黄疸、痢疾、水肿、翳、喉肿、痈肿疮毒、带状疱疹、跌打损伤。

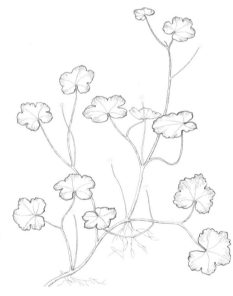

Hydrocotyle sibthorpioides Lam. is a kind of grass that can often be found in grassland, wetland and ditch, it is a common herbal medicine around us. Yunnan people also call it Potongqian, Poxian, Xiancao, Mantianxing, Feifengcao and Jichangcai. The whole plant of *Hydrocotyle sibthorprides* Lam. and Hydrocotyle sibthorpioides Lam. Var. Batrachium (Hance) Hand. -Mazz. ex Shan can be used as medicine. It is distributed in provinces of the south of the Yangtze River in China. As long as the grass is rubbed, it will give off a special smell and the whole herb of the umbelliferae creeping plant can be used as medicine. It tastes pungent and slight bitter with cold property. It has the effects of clearing heat and draining dampness, resolving toxin and dispersing swelling. It is mainly used to treat icterus, dysentery, edema, corneal opacity, sore swollen throat, carbuncle, herpes zoster and traumatic injuries.

30.（深）山酢浆草 *Oxalis griffithit* Edgew. & Hook. f.

　　雨季的昆明随处可见这种野草，摘下叶子放到嘴里一嚼，味道酸酸的，它就是酢浆草科酢浆草属的多年生草本植物深山酢浆草。和匍匐生的酢浆草相比，其植株要比酢浆草大得多，而且叶子的形状也和酢浆草有明显的区别。深山酢浆草也是我们身边的一种草药，其全草都可以入药，味酸、微辛，性平，具有活血化瘀、清热解毒的功效，用于治疗劳伤疼痛、麻风、无名肿毒、癫子、疥、癣、小儿鹅口疮、烫火伤、蛇咬伤、脱肛、跌打扭伤。

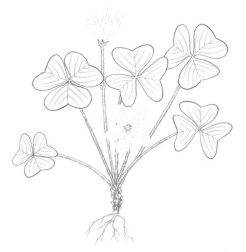

This kind of weed can be seen everywhere in Kunming during the rainy season, its leaves taste sour, is a perennial herb of Oxalisacetosella L., which belongs to Oxalidaceae genus and Oxalis family. Compared with the creeping oxalis, its roots and stems are much larger than the creeping woodsorrel, and the shape of the leaves also have obvious differences. Its whole plant can be used as herbal medicine, and it tastes sour and slight pungent with mild property. It has the effects of promoting blood circulation to remove blood stasis as well as clearing heat and removing toxicity. And it is mainly used to treat internal lesion caused by overexertion, leprosy, innominate inflammatory of unknown origin, favus, scabies, tinea, children thrush, burn and scald, snake bite, rectocele and traumatic injuries.

31. 滇龙胆草

Gentiana rigescens Franch.

滇龙胆草是龙胆草科多年生的草本植物，主要分布在四川、贵州、云南、广西和湖南，云南人会把它当作龙胆草来使用。其肉质须根是中医的入药部位，其味苦，性寒。由于滇龙胆味苦性寒，所以脾胃虚寒或者阴虚津伤的患者一般不宜使用。

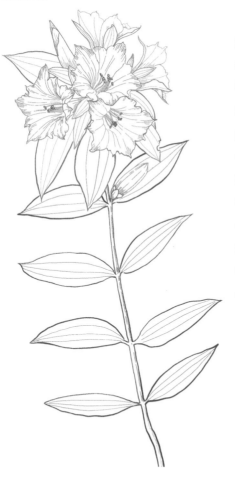

Gentiana rigescens Franch. is a perennial herb of the gentian family and mainly distributed in Sichuan, Guizhou, Yunnan, Guangxi and Hunan. Yunnan people often use it as a gentian root. Its fleshy fibrous roots can be used as herbal medicine and it tastes bitter with cold property. Patients with deficiency-cold in spleen and stomach or Yin deficiency and impairment of fluid are not suitable to use it due to its cold and bitter property.

32. 香叶天竺葵

Pelargonium hortarum L. H. Bailey

牻牛儿科植物香叶天竺葵是一种香气浓烈的花卉，和天竺葵是同科同属植物，但是天竺葵有一种令人难以接受的味道，而香叶天竺葵却香气四溢，味道令人神清气爽。它不仅有美化环境的效果，还可以净化空气、驱赶蚊虫，所以人们比较喜欢把它放在室内，并把它叫作驱蚊草。

Pelargonium hortarum L. H. Bailey is a kind of flower with strong fragrance and a plant has the same family and genus to geranium, and geranium has an unpleasant smell. While *Pelargonium hortarum* L. H. Bailey, has overflowing fragrance and it tastes refreshing, therefore, it not only has the effect of beautifying the environment, but also can purify the air and repel mosquitoes. So people prefer to put it indoors and call it Mozzie buster.

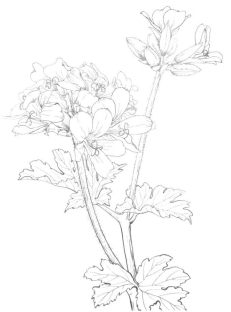

香叶天竺葵也是我们身边的一种草药，它的中药名就叫香叶。入药部位是它的茎叶，味辛，性温，无毒。全草治风湿，叶治疝气。

Pelargonium hortarum L. H. Bailey is also a herb around us, and its Chinese medicine name is Xiangye. The stem and leaves of this Geraniaceae plant are used in traditional Chinese medicine, it tastes pungent with mild property and non-toxic. Its whole plant can be used to treat rheumatism and its leaves can cure hernia.

33. 三棱草(碎米莎草)　　*Cyperus iria* L.

　　三棱草是莎草科植物碎米莎草的带根全草。主要分布于华东、华南、西南各地。作为一种常见的草药，三棱草在《中华本草》和《中药大词典》当中都有详细的记载。它味辛，性平，归肺经，无毒，具有解表透疹，催生之功效，常用于小儿痧疹不出，妇人难产。

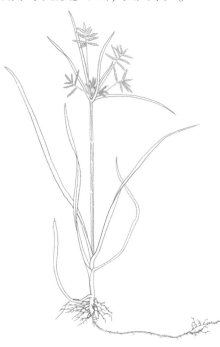

Cyperus iria L. is a herb of the sedge family of Cyperus iria Linn, it mainly distributes in east China, south China and southwest China. As a common herbal medicine, *Bdboschoenus mavitimus*(L.) Palla in Hauier & Brand was detailly recorded in *Chinese Materia Medica* and *Dictionary of Chinese Materia Medica*, it tastes pungent with mild property, attributes to lung meridian and non-toxic. It has the effects of relieving exterior syndrome for promoting eruption and hastening child delivery. It is often used for acute filthy of children with eruption difficulty and difficult labor.

34. 一点红   *Emilia sonchifolia*（L.）DC in Wight

一点红是菊科一年生或多年生草本植物，分布于陕西、江苏、浙江、江西、福建、湖北、湖南、广东、广西、四川、贵州及云南等地。只要你走路稍加留意，就会发现身边就开着这样的小花，花型精致小巧，而且颜色鲜艳，所以人们叫它一点红。

Emilia sonchifolia (L.) DC in Wight is an annual or perennial herb of the composite family and it mainly distributes in Shaanxi, Jiangsu, Zhejiang, Jiangxi, Fujian, Hubei, Hunan, Guangdong, Guangxi, Sichuan, Guizhou and Yunnan. You may find the small and delicate flowers with bright color around you as long as you pay attention to the roadsides when you are walking, so people call it Yidianhong.

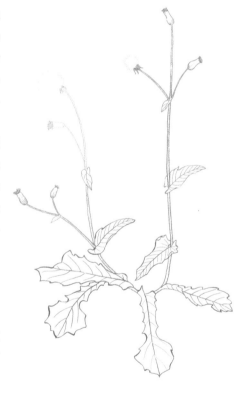

它也是我们身边的一种草药，它全草都可以入药。味苦，性凉，无毒，有清热解毒，散瘀消肿之功效，用于治疗上呼吸道感染、口腔溃疡、肺炎、乳腺炎、肠炎、菌痢、尿路感染、疮疖痈肿、湿疹、跌打损伤。

Emilia sonchifolia(L.) DC in Wight is also a herbal medicine around us and its whole plant can be used as herbal medicine, it tastes bitter with cold property and non-toxic. It has the effects of clearing heat and detoxicating, removing blood stasis and promoting the subsidence of swelling. It is mainly used to treat upper respiratory tract infection, oral ulcer, pneumonia, mastitis, enteritis, dysentery, urinary tract infection, sore and furuncle, eczema and traumatic injuries.

35. 格桑花（秋英） *Cosmos bipinnatus* Cav.

每到中秋前后，云南随处可见一种艳丽的花朵，它总是成片成片地盛开于山坡路边和公路两旁，把秋天的云南装扮得更加多彩。在滇西北高原地区，老百姓把它叫作格桑花；在滇中一带，人们则把它叫作波斯菊或者是国庆花，因为它盛开的时候正是国庆节。这种花实际上就是菊科秋英属一二年生草本植物秋英，又称波斯菊，入药部位是花或者全草。秋英原产于墨西哥，现在中国的大部分省区都有栽种，它的花朵不仅赏心悦目，同时也是我们身边的一种草药。在《全国中草药汇编》里也叫它痢疾草，味辛，性凉，具有清热解毒，化湿的功效，主治急、慢性痢疾，目赤肿痛，外用治痈疮肿毒。

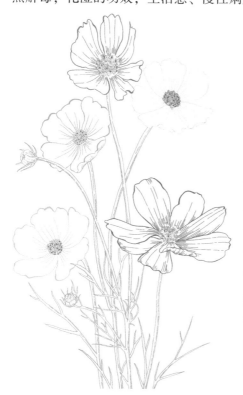

There are lots of gorgeous flowers blooming on the hillsides and road-sides around the Mid-Autumn Festival in every corner of Yunnan, which dresses up the Yunnan with colorful and magnificent view in Autumn. In the northwest plateau area of Yunnan, people call it Gesang flower, and Cosmos bipinnatus or National Day flower in the central area of Yunnan, because it will be in full bloom during the National Day. Actually, it is a year or two herb of Compositae and Cosmos, also known as *Cosmos bipinnatus* Cav and its flower or whole plant can be used as medicinal herbs. *Cosmos bipinnatus* Cav is native to Mexico and is now grown in most provinces and regions of China, its flowers are not only pleasing to the eyes, but also herbal medicine around us. It is called Lijicao in *National Compilation of Chinese Herbal Medicine*, it tastes pungent with cold property and has the effects of clearing heat, removing toxicity and dissipating dampness. It is often used to treat acute and chronic dysentery, sore red swollen eyes and external use to treat carbuncle, sore and swollen boils.

36. 大丽菊（大丽花）

Dahlia pinnata Cav.

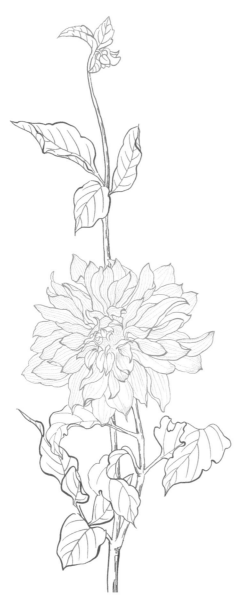

大丽菊，学名叫大丽花，菊科大丽花属多年生草本植物。由于它易栽易活，而且不需要特殊的护理，所以人们比较喜欢把它栽种于庭院。这种原产于墨西哥的花卉，如今在云南甚至全国各省区都有栽种。只需把它的根块埋于土中，不久就可以长出幼苗，由于它的花色艳丽夺目，所以很受人欢迎。

It is the perennial herb of Compositae and Dahlia Cav., also known as *Dahlia pinnata* Cav. in Mexico. It is now grown in Yunnan and even in all provinces and regions of China, people prefer to plant it in their yards due to it is easy growing and no special care is required, just bury its roots in the soil and it can soon grow seedlings, it is very popular because of its gorgeous and eye-catching colors.

大丽菊也是我们身边的一味草药，作为药用植物，其中药名就叫大丽菊，入药部位为其植物的块根。味辛、甘，性平，具有清热解毒，散瘀止痛的功效，主治腮腺炎、龋齿疼痛、无名肿毒、跌打损伤等病症。

Its tuberous roots can be used as herbal medicine and its medicinal name is Daliju. It tastes pungent and sweet with mild property and has the effects of clearing heat, removing toxicity, dissipating blood stasis to relieve pain. It is often used to treat mumps, caries pain, innominate inflanunatory of unknown origin and traumatic injuries.

37. 长鞭红景天

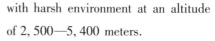

Rhodiola fastigiata（HK. f. et Thoms.）S. H. Fu

长鞭红景天是景天科红景天属多年生草本植物。分布于西藏、云南、四川，其生长环境十分恶劣，多在海拔 2500—5400 米的山坡石上。

It is the perennial herb of Crassulaceae and Rhodiola, and mostly distributed in Xizang, Yunnan, Sichuan, growing on the rocky hillsides with harsh environment at an altitude of 2, 500—5, 400 meters.

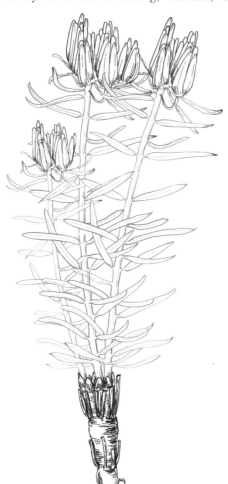

作为一种中药，其中药名就叫长鞭红景天，其味甘、微苦，性温，具有补血调经，养阴的功效，用于治疗月经不调、阴虚潮热、头晕目眩、妇女虚劳、骨蒸劳热等病症。

Its medicinal name is rhodiola fastigiate and it tastes sweet and slightly bitter with mild property. It has the effects of replenishing blood and regulating menstruation as well as nourishing Yin. It is often used to treat irregular menstruation, hot flush due to Yin deficiency, dizziness, women consumptive disease and hectic fever due to Yin-deficiency.

38. 香薷（石香薷）
Mosla chinensis Maxim.

这种长在花坛里的野草实际上是一味中药：香薷。用手揉搓它的茎叶和花穗，能够散发出一股强烈的芳香气味，所以人们又把它叫作香菜。它为唇形科石荠苧属植物，学名叫石香薷，其入药部位为全草或者地上部分。

The weed growing in the flower bed is actually an herbal medicine named Xiangru, it will give off a strong aromatic fragrance when its stems, leaves and flower buds are being rubbed, so it is also called Xiangcai. Its whole herb or above ground parts can be used as herbal medicine.

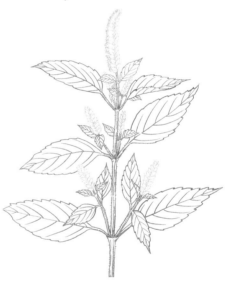

味辛，性微温，归肺、脾、胃经，具有发汗解表、化湿和中、利水消肿的功效，主治风寒感冒、水肿、脚气。它鲜嫩的茎叶是可以拿来当菜吃的，每年夏秋季，香薷开花的季节，就是我们采收的季节，将其采割、洗净、晒干以后就可以入药。

It tastes pungent with minor mild property and belongs to lung, spleen and stomach meridian. It has the effects of inducing sweat and dispelling exogenous e-vils, removing dampness for regulating stomach and inducing diuresis to alleviate edema. It can be used to treat wind-cold, edema and dermatophytosis. In addition, its tender stems and leaves can be eaten as vegetables. Harvest them during blooming season in summer and autumn and use them as medicine after being washed clean and dried in the sun.

39. 毛莨铁线莲

Clematis ranunculoides Franch

在昆明市郊的梁王山上，常常能看到一种植物，当地很多人把它叫作威灵仙，它其实是毛莨科铁线莲属多年生草质藤本植物，叫作毛莨铁线。毛莨铁线莲分布于云南西北部、四川西南部、广西西北部及贵州西南部。

This kind of plants can be found in the Liangwang Mountains at the outskirts

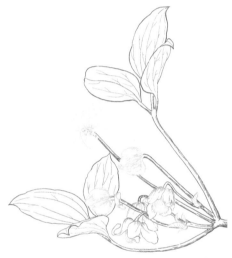

of Kunming and it is called Weilingxian by local people. actually it is the perennial grassy vine of Ranunculaceae and Clematis L. , and known as *Clematis ranunculoides* Franch. It is distributed in northwest Yunnan, southwest Sichuan, northwest Guangxi and southwest Guizhou.

作为药用植物，其中药名就叫毛莨铁线，其味苦、淡、微辛，性微寒，具有清热解毒、利尿、祛瘀通络的功效，主治疮痈疖肿，乳腺炎，水肿，小便不利，癃闭，跌打损伤等病症。

Its medicinal name is Maogentiexianlian and it tastes bitter, bland and slightly pungent with minor cold property. It has the effects of clearing heat, removing toxicity, inducing urine and removing blood stasis to regulate collaterals. It is often used to treat sore and swollen boils, mammitis, edema, inhibited urination, retention of urine and traumatic injuries.

云南的彝族把它叫灯笼衣，临床上主要用它的根来入药，具有利尿和解毒的功效，可以治疗云翳、小儿疳积、手足麻木、痞块以及消化不良和脓疮。

Yi people in Yunnan call it Denglongyi and use its roots as medicine for its urine induction and toxicity removing effects, which can cure corneal opacity, infantile malnutrition, numb hands and feet, lump in the abdomen, indigestion and abscess.

40. 千针万线草

Stellaria yunnanensis Franch

千针万线草主要分布在我国的云南、贵州、四川和西藏，是石竹科繁缕属植物，以其根作为入药部位。它不像其他中药一样的苦涩，而是一味名副其实的山珍美味，云南很多当地人把它作为一味补药，用于食疗补虚。用千针万线草的根须炖肉吃，不仅口味甘甜还有一股特殊的香味。

It is the herb of Caryophyllaceae and Stellaria, and mainly distributed in southwest provinces of China and Xizang. Its roots can be used as herbal medicine and they are not as bitter as other traditional Chinese medicine, actually, it is a veritable mountain delicacy and Yunnan people regard it as a tonic for diet therapy to supplement deficiency. In addition, stew its roots with meat, the soup tastes sweet and has a very special fragrance.

千针万线草，味甘，性平，归肝、脾、肾经，具有健脾养血、补肝益肾、消肿的作用，主治贫血、精神短少、头晕心慌、耳鸣眼花、潮热、遗精、月经不调、带下、骨折、乳腺炎等病症。

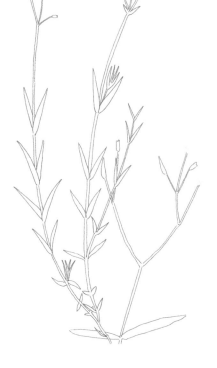

Its medicinal name is Qianzhenwanxiancao and it tastes sweet with mild property, belongs to liver, spleen and kidney meridian. It has the effects of invigorating spleen and nourishing blood, tonifying liver and kidney as well as removing swelling. It is mainly used to treat anemia, lassitude, dizziness and panic, tinnitus and dizziness, hectic fever, emission, irregular menstruation, morbid leucorrhea, fractures and mastitis.

41. 无患子
Sapindus saponaria L.

　　无患子是身材高大的落叶乔木，是无患子科无患子属木本植物，分布于我国华东、中南和西南地区。无患子又叫肥珠子、木患子、桂圆肥皂、圆肥皂、洗手子。它的根、树皮、嫩枝叶、果肉和果核都可以入药。在云南，无患子常被当地人用来洗衣服、洗头，要是有的人皮肤长疮疖，他们会把无患子的根皮挖回家煮水来洗。

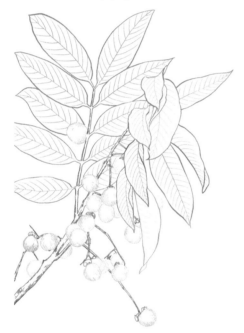

It is a tall and big deciduous woody arbor of Sapindaceae and Soapberry and distributed in east China, south central and southwest China. It is also called Feizhuzi, Muhuanzi, Guiyuanfeizao, Yuanfeizao, Xishouzi, and its root, bark, tender branches and leaves, flesh and pit can be used as herbal medicine. It is often used by the Yunnan locals to wash clothes and hair, and if someone has sore boil, people will dig its root and boil it to wash the skin.

　　中医常用的无患子饮片，其实是其种子。无患子，味苦、辛，性寒，入心、肺经，小毒。具有清热、祛痰、消积、杀虫的功效，主治喉痹肿痛、肺热咳喘、音哑、食滞、疳积、蛔虫腹痛、滴虫性阴道炎、癣疾、肿毒等病症。

In fact, the decoction pieces of Wuhuanzi are the seeds of it. It has minor toxicity and tastes bitter and pungent with cold property, belongs to heart and lung meridian. It has the effects of clearing heat, eliminating phlegm, removing food retention and killing insects. It is often used to treat sore and swollen throat, dyspnea and cough due to lung-heat, muting, dyspepsia, malnutritional stagnation, abdominal pain caused by roundworm, trichomonas vaginitis, ringworm disease and pyogenic infections.

42. 板蓝根（菘蓝）

Isatis tinctoria L.

菘蓝是十字花科菘蓝属二年生草本植物。菘蓝在我国的大部分省区都有种植，在云南的一些菜市场上，我们经常可以见到它的叶子作为蔬菜在售卖。它干燥的根和叶就是中药板蓝根和大青叶。

It is the biennial herb of Cruciferae and Isatis L. and it is grown in most provinces of China. We can often see its leaves sold as vegetables in some vegetable markets in Yunnan, and its dried roots and leaves can be used as herbal medicine, also known as radix isatidis and folium isatidis.

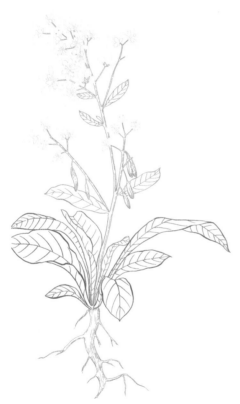

其味苦，性寒，归心、胃经，具有清热解毒、凉血、利咽的功效，主治外感发热、温病初起、咽喉肿痛、温毒发斑、疟腮、丹毒、痈肿疮毒等病症。

It tastes bitter with cold property and belongs to heart and stomach meridian. It has the effects of clearing heat, removing toxicity, cooling blood and relieving sore throat. It is often used to treat exogenous fever, onset of febrile disease, swollen sore throat, spot on the skin caused by warm-pathogenic, mumps, erysipelas, sore and swollen boils.

43. 蕨

Pteridium aquilinum voy. *latiusculum* (Desv.) Underw. ex A. Heller

蕨又叫蕨菜，为蕨科蕨属植物蕨的一个变种。它在我国的分布非常广泛，从南到北到处都有，云南各地山坡，甚至田间地头都可见到。除了是人们喜爱的野菜以外，它还是我们身边的一味草药。作为药用植物，其中药名就叫蕨，入药部位为叶，味甘，性寒，具有清热、利湿、止血、降气、化痰的功效，主治感冒发热、黄疸、痢疾、带下、噎膈、肺结核咳血、肠风便血、风湿痹痛等病症。

It is a variation of Pteridiaceae and Moorwort and widely distributed in China, it can be found on hillsides and even fields all over Yunnan. In addition to being people's favourite wild vegetables, it is also an herb around us and its medicinal name is Peteridium aquilinum. Its leaves taste sweet with cold property and it has the effects of clearing heat, eliminating dampness, stopping blood, depressing Qi and resolving phlegm. It is often used to treat cold and fever, jaundice, dysentery, leukorrhagia, dysphagia, pulmonary tuberculosis hemoptysis, hematochezia and rheumatic arthralgia.

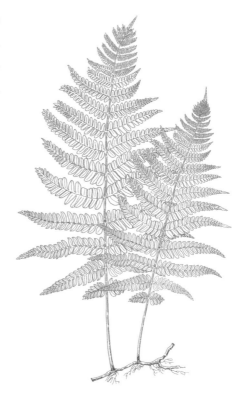

除了鲜嫩的叶可以入药以外，其根也可以入药。早在明代著名医家李时珍的《本草纲目》当中就有蕨根作为中药的记载，蕨根又叫蕨鸡根、小角和乌角，一般我们秋冬季将其采挖，洗净晒干就可以入药。蕨根味甘，性寒，无毒，具有清热利湿、平肝安神和解毒消肿的功效。

In addition to its tender leaves, its roots can also be used as medicine, which was recorded as early as in famous doctor Li Shizhen's *Compendium of Materia Medica* in the Ming Dynasty. It is also called Juejigen, Xiaojiao and Wujiao, its roots can be harvested in autumn and used as medicine after being washed clean and dried in the sun. It is nontoxic and tastes sweet with cold property, and has the effects of clearing heat and eliminating dampness, calming liver and relieving uneasiness of mind, removing toxicity and dispersing swelling.

44. 龙血树

Dracaena draco（L.）L.

龙血树，龙舌兰科龙血树属常绿乔木。龙血树全身是宝，据《全国中草药汇编》介绍，龙血树的根块可以直接入药，它的树脂就是大家熟知的血竭。在海南等地，也有把细枝龙血树的根须拿来做药的习惯，龙血树的根块味甘，性凉，具有润肝止咳、清热凉血的功效。

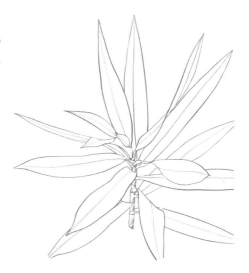

It is the evergreen arbor of Agavaceae and Dracaena, according to the *National Compilation of Chinese Herbal Medicine*, its whole plants are treasures and its root blocks can be directly used as medicine, and its resin is known as resina draconis. There is also a habit of using its root hair as medicine in Hainan and other places, its root blocks taste sweet with cold property and has the effects of moistening liver and relieving cough, clearing heat and cooling blood.

龙血树的叶子也是可以入药的，《云南省中药材标准》（2005 年版第三册）当中详细介绍了龙血树叶的性味归经和临床功效：龙血树叶，味淡、微涩，性平，具有清火解毒、除风消疮、活血化瘀、消肿止痛、续筋解骨的功效，可以用它来治疗贫血、产后体弱多病、心慌惊悸、胃脘疼痛、吐血、便血、泄泻、风湿性关节炎、肢体肿胀疼痛、腮腺炎、淋巴结炎、乳腺炎、乳腺囊性增生、肿瘤、癫痫、胸闷、心痛、消渴、外伤出血、跌打损伤、骨折等病症。

Yunnan Provincial Standard of Chinese Medicinal Materials（Volume 3, 2005 edition）illustrated in detail that its leaves can be used as medicine and it tastes bland, slightly astringent with mild property, and it has the effects of clearing heat and removing toxicity, eliminating wind evil and removing ulcer, promoting blood circulation to remove blood stasis, relieving swelling and pain, reinforcing tendons and setting fracture. It can be used to treat anemia, valetudinarianism after delivery, palpitation, epigastric pain, hematemesis, hematochezia, diarrhea, rheumatic arthritis, limb swelling and pain, mumps, lymphnoditis, mammitis, breast cystic hyperplasia, tumor, epilepsy, chest distress, cardiac pain, diabetes, traumatic bleeding, traumatic injuries and fractures.

45. 婆婆纳

Veronica polita Fries

婆婆纳为玄参科婆婆纳属植物。分布于西南、西北、华东、华中。婆婆纳属植物是一个庞大的家族，在我国就有60多种，记载入药的多达27种。作为药用植物，其中药名就叫婆婆纳，婆婆纳以全草入药。其味甘、淡，性凉，入肝、肾经，具有补肾强腰、解毒消肿的功效，常用于肾虚腰痛、疝气、睾丸肿痛、妇女白带、痈肿等病证。

It is the plant of Scrophulariaceae and Veronica and distributes in southwest, northwest, east and central China. It is a huge family of plants and there are more than 60 varieties in China, and as many as 27 kinds of them have been listed as medicine. Its whole plant can be used as medicine and its medicinal name is Veronica didyma Tenore. It tastes sweet and bland with cold property, belongs to liver and kidney meridian, and it has the effects of tonifying kidney and strengthening waist, removing toxicity and eliminating swelling. It is often used to treat kidney deficiency and lumbar pain, hernia, testis swollen and pain, leucorrhea and abscess.

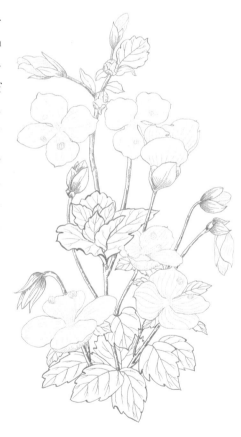

近些年来，国内外学者对婆婆纳的药用活性进行了深入的研究，首先婆婆纳属植物有明显的抗氧化活性，由于它们普遍含有多酚羟基的苯乙醇苷和环烯蜜醚萜苷类化合物质，这些物质都具有良好的清除自由基和抗氧

化活性。有学者从阿拉伯婆婆纳当中分离出一种显化黄酮糖苷，这种物质有很强的清除自由基活性作用。

Scholars at home and abroad have conducted in-depth studies on the medicinal activities of Veronica didyma Tenore in recent years and found that Verona plants have obvious antioxidant activities due to their common compounds containing polyphenol hydroxyl phenylethanol glycosides and iridoid glycosides, which have good free radical scavenging and antioxidant activities. In addition, some scholars have distracted a manifest flavonoid glycoside from Arabic Veronica persica, which has a strong DPPH clearance activity.

婆婆纳属植物还有明显的抗癌活性，阿拉伯婆婆纳的甲醇提取物对KB上皮癌细胞和B16黑色素瘤，具有明显的抑制作用。其细胞毒活性成分集中于氯仿萃取部分，而且其作用强度随着给药剂量的增加而增强。研究还表明，婆婆纳属植物当中提取的水漫晶总磺酮对前列腺炎有明显的抑制作用，同时它还具有抑制模型动物前列腺增生的作用。

Furthermore, Arabic Veronica persica also has significant anticancer activity and its methanol extract has obvious inhibitory effect on KB epithelial cancer cells and B16 melanoma, and its cytotoxic active components were concentrated in chlorine spinning extraction and the strength of the action strengthened with the increase of the dose. Research also shows that its total sulfosterone extraction has obvious inhibitory effect on prostatitis and it also has inhibitory effect on prostatic hyperplasia in model animals.

46. 云木香　　*Aucklandia costus* Falc

　　木香一般分为广木香、云木香和川木香，我们常把从印度等地进口的木香和广东产的木香叫广木香，把主产于云南、广西的木香称为云木香，而主产于四川、西藏的木香则叫川木香。三者在功效上没有太大的区别。云木香是菊科云木香属多年生高大草本植物。作为药用植物，其中药名就叫云木香，入药部位为根，其味辛、苦，性温。具有行气止痛、温中和胃的功效，临床上常用于治疗胸腹胀满、呕吐、泄泻、痢疾、里急后重等病症。

Aucklandia costus Falc is generally divided into costus root, Aucklandia costus and common vladimiria root, and aucklandia imported from India and Guangdong Aucklandia called costus root, Aucklandia mainly produced in Yunnan and Guangxi is called Aucklandia costus, and the aucklandia grown in Sichuan and Xizang is called common vladimiria root, and there is no much efficacy differences among them. Aucklandia costus is the tall and perennial plant

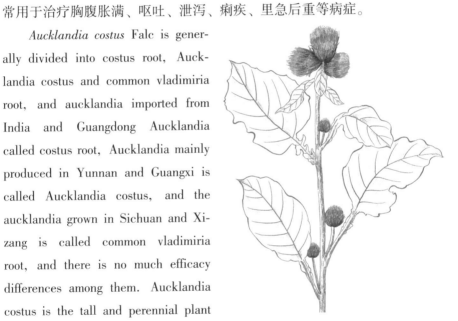

of Compositae and Aucklandia. Its roots can be used as herbal medicine and its medicinal name is Aucklandia costus. It tastes pungent and bitter with mild property, and it has the effects of promoting Qi circulation to relieve pain and warming the stomach, and it is often used to treat chest and abdominal distention, vomiting, diarrhoea, dysentery and tenesmus.

　　由于木香性温，所以阴虚内热者不要使用。

Patient suffers from internal heat due to Yin deficiency is not suitable to use Aucklandia costus due to its warm property.

47. 两面针

Zanthoxylum nitidum（Roxb.）DC.

两面针是芸香科花椒属植物，在我国南方的大部分省区都有分布，人们又把它叫作两背针、双面针、叶下穿针、入地金牛、红心刺刁根等。作为药用植物，其中药名就叫两面针，它干燥的根是中医的入药部位，其味苦、辛，性平，有小毒，具有活血化瘀、行气止痛、祛风通络、解毒消肿的功效，在临床上常用于治疗跌打损伤、胃痛、牙痛、风湿痹痛、虫舌咬伤等病症，外用可以治疗烧烫伤。

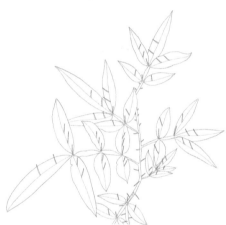

It is the plant of Rutaceae and Zanthoxylum, distributes in most of the southern provinces of China and it is also called Liangmianzhen, Shuangmianzhen, Yexiachuanzhen, Rudijinniu and Hongxincidiaogen. Its dried roots can be used as herbal medicine and its medicinal name is Zanthoxylum nitidum. It has minor toxicity and tastes bitter, pungent with mild property, and it has the effects of promoting blood circulation to remove blood stasis, promoting Qi circulation to relieve pain, dispelling wind and removing obstruction in the meridians, resolving toxin and dispersing swelling.

使用两面针可以煎汤内服，可以研磨调敷或者水煎洗外用，由于两面针有小毒，所以不可以过量使用，也不能和酸味的食物同时食用。

Take its decoction orally, apply its grinded power or wash with its decocted soup externally. It cannot be used over dose, nor can it be eaten with sour food simultaneously.

48. 土茯苓

Smilax glabra Roxb.

在云南的郊区路边、林下、山坡，到处都可以见到这种植物——土茯苓。它和菝葜很相似，只不过它的叶子细长而菝葜的叶子宽大。菝葜的茎秆有小刺，而土茯苓的茎秆是光滑的。

Smilax glabra Roxb. can be easily found on the roadsides, under forests and slopes in the suburbs of Yunnan. It looks like Chinaroot greenbrier, while its leaves are long and slender with smooth stems, chinaroot greenbrier's leaves are big and wide with small thorns on the stems.

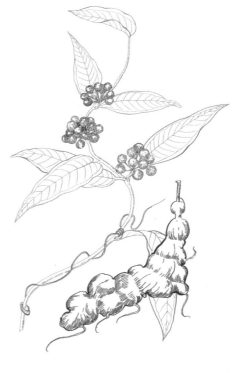

土茯苓是菝葜科菝葜属植物，主要在我国长江以南分布，在甘肃等部分北方省区也有分布。作为药用植物，其中药名就叫土茯苓，它的根茎是中医的入药部位。秋冬季将其采挖洗净，切片晒干以后就可以入药。其味甘、淡，性平，具有清热除湿、泄浊解毒、通利关节的功效，在临床上常用于治疗梅毒、淋浊、泄泻、筋骨挛痛、痈肿、瘰疬、瘿瘤等病证。肝肾阴虚者一定要慎重使用。

It is the plant of Smilacaceae and Smilax and mainly distributes in south of Yangtze River and some northern provinces in Gansu. Its rhizome can be used as herbal medicine and its medicinal name is Smilax Glabra. Harvest its rhizome in autumn and winter, and use them as medicine after being washed clean, sliced into pieces and dried in the sun. It tastes sweet and bland with mild property, and it has the effects of clearing heat and removing dampness, expelling turbidity and removing toxicity, easing joint movement. It is often used to treat syphilis, stranguria with turbid discharge, diarrhea, muscle and bone clonus pain, abscess, crewels, goiter and tumor clinically.

土茯苓是临床上常用的一味中药，现在药理研究也特别多。首先土茯苓具有明显的抗炎镇痛作用，其作用的部分是土茯苓当中含有的植物甾醇类物质，植物甾醇的物质成分比较复杂，但是其中有不少组分具有消除人体中的炎症的作用，并且可以促进伤口的愈合。

Smilax glabra Roxb. is a common traditional Chinese medicine in clinical practice and there are many pharmacological researches on it, while patient with liver and kidney Yin deficiency should use it with caution. Firstly, phytosterols contained in smilax glabra have distinctive antiphlogistic and analgesia effects, although the composition of phytosterols is complex in smilax glabra, many of these components have the effects of eliminating inflammation in the body and can promote wound healing.

另外土茯苓具有明显的免疫调节作用，这一功能与土茯苓当中含有的黄酮中的落新妇苷息息相关，现代研究已经证明，落新妇苷是一种常见的对于免疫细胞具有免疫调节作用的物质。大量研究证明，土茯苓对于人体肿瘤具有非常明显的作用，有学者用土茯苓醇提取物进行体外实验，证明它对宫颈癌的疗效是显著的。对某种类型的宫颈癌，癌细胞的抑制率可以达到90%以上。另有学者研究发现，土茯苓当中的活性物质对黄曲霉毒素 B_1 引起的大鼠肝癌，有显著的治疗效果。

Secondly, astilbin in flavonoids contained in smilax glabra has obvious immune regulation effect and the modern research shows that astilbin has an immunomodulatory effect on immune cells. Furthermore, a large number of studies have proved that smilax glabra has a very obvious effect on human tumors, and some scholars have carried out in vitro experiments with its extract, proved that it has a significant effect on cervical cancer, and the inhibition rate of cancer cells can reach more than 90%. In addition, some scholars also found that active substance in smilax glabra has remarkable therapeutic effect on liver cancer in rats caused by aflatoxin B_1.

研究证明，土茯苓对缓解动脉粥样硬化症具有很好的疗效，土茯苓对下腔静脉血栓也有很好的治疗效果，这大大地开拓了我们治疗心血管系统疾病方面的思路。

Studies have proved that smilax glabra has a good effect on alleviating atherosclerosis and inferior vena cava thrombosis, which offers a lot of new thinking on how to treat cardiovascular diseases.

土茯苓还有保肝护肝的作用，它的水提取物对肝损伤具有明显的治疗效果，此外，还有很多关于土茯苓治疗高尿酸血症和镇咳、祛痰等作用的研究报道，都为我们临床使用土茯苓打开了新的视野。

In addition, smilax glabra's water extract has obvious therapeutic effect on liver injury, so it also has the role of protecting liver. Furthermore, there are also many studies on the effect of smilax glabra in the treatment of hyperuricemia, antitussive and expectorant, which have opened a new vision for our clinical use of smilax glabra.

49. 胡椒木

Zanthoxylum'Odorum

胡椒木是芸香科花椒属的长粒灌木植物。揉搓它的枝叶，能够散发出一股浓烈的芳香气味，有如胡椒的香气，所以人们把它叫作胡椒木。

It is the long grain shrub plant of Rutaceae and Zanthoxylum, it will give off a strong aroma smelling like pepper when rub its branches and leaves, so it is called Zanthoxylum piperitum.

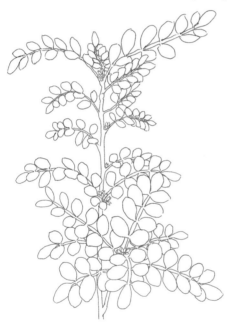

胡椒木不仅是常见的绿化植物，也是我们身边的一味草药。作为药用植物，其中药名就叫胡椒木，它的根是入药部位。其味辛，性温，具有温中、下气、消痰和解毒的功效，可以用它来治疗寒痰食积，也就是脾胃阳虚导致的痰湿内壅、消化不良等病症。还可以治疗脘腹冷痛、反胃、呕吐清水、泄泻、冷痢，也就是下痢日久伤及脾阳的病症。胡椒木由于性温，所以阴虚燥热的患者是不宜使用的。

Zanthoxylum piperitum is not only a common green plant, but also an herb around us. Its roots can be used as herbal medicine and its medicinal name is Zanthoxylum piperitum. It tastes pungent with warm property and has the effects of warming the middle warmer, descending Qi, eliminating phlegm and removing toxicity. It can be used to treat obstructed phlegm and dampness caused by spleen-stomach Yang deficiency, indigestion, stomach and abdomen cold pain, regurgitation, vomiting of clear water, diarrhea, cold dysentery and spleen Yang damage. Patients with Yin deficiency and dry heat are not suitable to use Zanthoxylum piperitum due to its warm property.

50. 小蓟（刺儿菜）

Cirstum arvense var. integrifolium Wimm. & Grab.

小蓟，学名刺儿菜，菊科蓟属多年生草本植物。作为药用植物，其中药名就叫小蓟，其地上部分为入药部位，其味甘、苦，性凉，具有凉血、止血、散瘀、解毒、消痈的功效。

Cirstum arvense var. integrifolium Wimm. & Grab. is the perennial herb of Compositae and Cirsium, it is also called Ciercai and its above ground plant can be used as herbal medicine and its medicinal name is called Cirsium setosum. It tastes sweet and bitter with cold property, and it has the effects of cooling blood, stopping bleeding, dispersing stasis, removing toxicity and eliminating carbuncle.

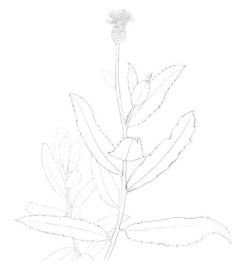

小蓟和大蓟在功效上非常相似，除了凉血、止血以外，大蓟的解毒消痈功效要强于小蓟。小蓟除了止血以外还有利尿的功能，由于小蓟性凉，所以体质虚寒的患者要慎重使用。

Cirsium setosum and Circium japonicum are very similar in efficacy, in addition to cooling blood and stopping bleeding, circium japonicum's detoxification and carbuncle elimination effect is stronger than circium setosum. In addition to blood stopping effect, circium setosum also has the effect of inducing urine, while people with cold and deficiency constitution should use it with caution.

51. 莪术（蓬莪术）

Curcuma phaeocaulis Valeton

蓬莪术，姜科姜黄属多年生草本植物。中医将其根茎称"莪术"，供药用。这种姜科植物主要分布在云南、广西、广东、福建、湖南和江浙一带。

Curcuma phaeocaulis Valeton is the perennial herb of Zingiberaceae and curcuma, its roots and stems are called curcuma phaeocaulis in traditional Chinese medicine, which is mainly distributed in Yunnan, Guangxi, Guangdong, Guangdong, Fujian, Hunan, Jiangsu and Zhejiang provinces.

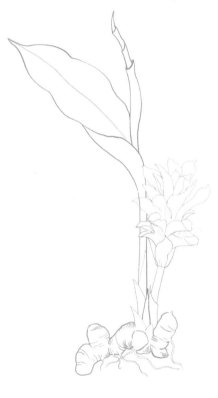

作为药用植物，其中药名就叫莪术，中医对莪术的传统认识是：其味辛、苦，性温，归肝、脾经，具有行气破血，消积止痛的功效，常用于血气心痛、饮食积滞、脘腹胀痛、血滞经闭、痛经、癥瘕痞块、跌打损伤等病症。云南著名的傣医艾罕丹认为傣医对莪术的临床使用范围要比中医广得多。据《中国傣药志》记载，莪术除了行气活血以外，它还具有清火解毒、敛疮生肌以及镇心安神的作用。可见同一种药在不同民族的用药经验中，使用范围是不完全相同的，值得我们深入研究，以不断地完善中医药学，这也是我们研究少数民族医药的意义所在。

Its medicinal name is curcuma phaeocaulis and tastes pungent, bitter with warm property, belongs to liver and spleen meridian. It has the effects of regulating Qi and activating blood circulation, eliminating accumulation and relieving pain. It is often used to treat heartache due to Qi and blood deficiency, food stagnation, stomach and abdomen distention and pain, amenorrhea due to stagnation of blood, dysmenorrhea, lumps, traumatic injuries. AI Handan, a famous Dai doctor in Yunnan, holds the view that. the clinical application of curcuma phaeo-aulis in Dai medicine is much wider than that in traditional Chinese medicine. According to *Annals of Chinese Dai Medicine*, in addition to functions of promoting Qi and blood circulation, it also has the effects of clearing heat and removing toxicity, healing up sore and promoting granulation as well as calming the heart and tranquilizing the mind. Therefore, it can be seen that the usage scope of the same medicine in the medical experience of different ethnic groups is not exactly the same, which is worth our in-depth study to continuously improve the Chinese medicine, that is also the significance of our research on ethnomedicine.

52. 路边姜   *Hedychium covonarium* J. könig in Retzius

路边姜，是多年生姜科姜花属植物姜花的根茎。该植物主要分布在我国的热带、亚热带地区，在云南的南部地区到处可见。

Hedychium covonarium J. könig in Retzius is the roots of perennial plant of Zingiberaceae and Hedychium Koenig, which is mainly distributed in tropical and subtropical areas of China, it can be found everywhere in the Southern areas of Yunnan.

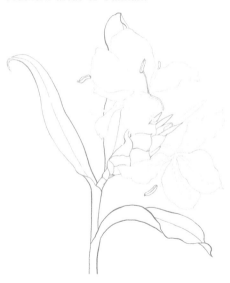

路边姜是姜花的根茎，云南的老百姓常把它的根茎挖回家当菜吃，这也是它的入药部位。作为药用植物，其中药名就叫路边姜，其味辛，性温，具有祛风散寒、温经止痛的功效。据《全国中草药汇编》介绍：姜花的果实也具有温中散寒的作用。其根状茎用于感冒、头痛身痛、风湿筋骨疼痛、跌打损伤、寒湿白带等病症。果用于胃脘胀闷、消化不良、寒滞作呕、胃腹微痛等病症。

Hedychium covonarium J. könig in Retzius is the roots of ginger flower, Yunnan people often dig its roots and take them as vegetable, they can also be used as herbal medicine and their medicinal name is Hedy chiumcoronarium. It tastes pungent with warm property and it has the effects of expelling wind evil and removing cold, warming the meridian to relieve pain. According to *National Compilation of Chinese Herbal Medicine*, the fruit of ginger flower also has the effects of warming the middle warmer and dispelling cold and its rhizome can be used to treat cold, head and body pain, rheumatic muscle pain, traumatic injuries, cold and damp leukorrhea. Its fruits can be used to treat stomach and abdomen distension and depression, indigestion, nausea due to cold stagnation and slight pain in the stomach.

53. 黄金菊 *Euryops pectinatus*（L.）Cass.

春天已过，满城的小黄花盛开，把凉爽的昆明春城点缀得更加漂亮。黄金菊不仅是美丽的花朵，也是我们身边的一种草药。

The small yellow flowers are in full blossom when the spring is over, which embellished the cool Kunming spring city more beautiful. *Euryops pectinatus*(L.) Cass. is a perennial herb of Compositae and Huangarong Chrysanthemum. It is not only a beautiful flower, but also a herb around us.

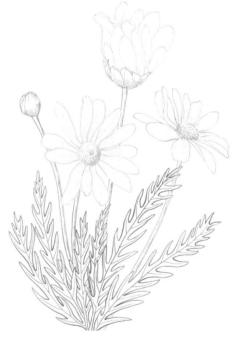

黄金菊又叫南非菊、翠菊木、银叶情人菊、银叶金木菊、疏黄菊、梳黄菊等，是菊科黄蓉菊属植物，中国各地均有栽培。作为药用植物，其中药名叫黄金菊根，性味甘、苦，性微寒，入肝经，具有平肝明目、疏风清热的功效。据《中华本草》介绍，其主治视物模糊，目赤肿痛，咽喉疼痛，外感风热或者风温初起引起的发热、头痛、眩晕等病症。

It is the plant of Compositae and Huangarong Chrysanthemum and it is cultivated all over China, also called Nanfeiju, Cuijumu, Yinyeqingrenju, Yinyejinmuju and Shuhuangju. Its medicinal name Huang jin ju gen and it tastes sweet and bitter with minor cold property, belongs to liver meridian. It has the effects of calming the liver and improving the eyesight, dispersing wind evil and clearing heat. According to *National Chinese Materia Medica*, it can be used to treat blurred vision, sore red swollen eyes, sore throats, wind-heat cold or fever, headache, dizziness and other symptoms caused by the initial onset of wind heat.

54. 苦楝树

Melia azedarach L.

 　　苦楝树的花不仅美丽芳香，还是我们身边的一种常见药用植物，其花、叶、果实、根皮均可入药。其树皮及根皮入药叫苦楝皮，其味苦，性寒，有毒，归肝、脾、胃经，具有杀虫，疗癣的功效，主治蛔虫病，蛲虫病，钩虫病，疥癣，湿疮等病症。由于其性味苦寒，所以体弱者、肝肾功能不全者、孕妇或者是脾胃虚寒者是不宜使用的。

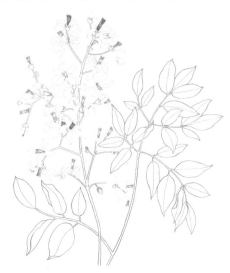

　　The flowers of Cortex Meliae are not only beautiful and fragrant, but also a common medicinal plant around us, its flowers, leaves, fruits and bark can be used as medicinal herb. Its dried bark and velamen are Kulianpi. It is toxic and tastes bitter with cold property, belongs to liver, spleen and meridian, and it has the effects of killing insects and curing ringworm. It can be used to treat ascariasis, enterobiasis, ancylostomiasis, mange and eczema. People with weak constitution and suffer from liver and kidney insufficiency as well as pregnant women or spleen and stomach deficiency cold are not suitable to use it due to its cold property.

　　苦楝树的花同样是一味中药，它的中药名叫苦楝花或者是楝花，其味苦，性寒，具有清热、除湿、杀虫、止痒的功效。楝花一般外用，可以研磨后或者是捣烂后敷在患处。

　　Its flowers can also be used as herbal medicine and its medicinal name is Kulianhua or Lianhua, which tastes bitter with cold property and has the effects of clearing heat, eliminating dampness, killing insects and relieving itching. It is generally used externally and can be ground or mashed then applied to the affected area.

　　苦楝树的叶也可以入药，它的中药名叫苦楝叶或者叫楝叶，其味苦，性寒，具有清热、燥湿、杀虫、止痒和行气止痛的功效，临床上使用楝叶多为外用，可以煎水外洗，也可捣烂外敷。

　　Its leaves can also be used as herbal medicine and its medicinal name is Kulianye or Lianye. It tastes bitter with cold property and has the effects of clearing heat, eliminating dampness, killing insects and promoting Qi circulation to relieve pain. It is often used externally by washing its decocted water or applying it on the affected area after being mashed.

55. 朱顶红

Hippeastrum vittatum（L'Her.）Hevb.

朱顶红，石蒜科朱顶红属植物。在中国是最为常见的花卉，它不仅可以作为花卉观赏，它的鳞茎也是我们身边的一味草药。这种原产于中南美洲的植物，在我国几乎到处都可以栽种，到处可见。

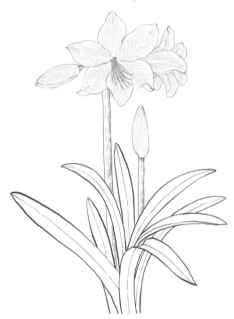

Hippeastrum vittatum(Kev-Gawl.) Hevb. is the plant of Litholiaceae and Hippeastrum, which is the most common flower in China and it can not only be used as ornamental plant, but its bulbs are also herbal medicine around us. It is native to Central and South America, it is now widely planted in China.

据《中华本草》介绍，它的鳞茎可入药，其中药名就叫朱顶红，其味辛，性温，具有清热解毒的功效。朱顶红作为中药使用是不能内服的，只能外用。

According to *Chinese Herbal Medicine*, its bulbs can be used as herbal medicine and its medicinal name is hippeastrum vittatum. It tastes pungent with warm property and it has the effects of clearing heat and removing toxicity. It can only be used externally.

56. 干檀香（沙针）

Dsyvis lanceolata Hochst. & Steud.

干檀香从前是老百姓上山挖这种树的树疙瘩来烤火的，因为其烧起来有一股特殊的清香，所以老百姓都把它叫作香疙瘩。这种小乔木或者灌木，实际上是檀香科沙针属的沙针或其变种豆瓣香树的全株植物。它主要分布在云南、广西、四川、贵州、西藏等西部地区，它的中药名叫干檀香，也有人叫它地檀香、小青皮、小清香、土檀香和山苏木。其药用价值在《中药大词典》《中华本草》和《全国中草药汇编》当中都有详细的记载：它的叶具有祛瘀血、解毒疮的作用，一般煎水外洗、研末外撒或者捣烂外敷。

The lump on the trees were used to be ignited to get warm by people, they called it fragrant lump due to its special fragrance when burning. It is actually the whole plant of Santalaceae and OsyrisLinn of Osyris wightiana Wall. ex Wight or its variant Osyris wightiana Wall. ex Wight var. rotundifolia(Tam), which is mainly dis-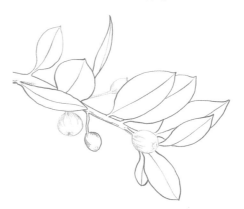tributed in Yunnan, Guangxi, Sichuan, Guizhou and Xizang, its medicinal name is dried sandalwood and people also call it Ditangxinag, Xiaoqingpi, Xiaoqingxiang, Tutangxiang and Shansumu. Its medicinal value was recorded in detail in *Dictionary of Chinese Materia Medica*, *Chinese Herbal Medicine* and *National Compilation of Chinese Herbal Medicine* that its leaves have the effects of removing blood stasis and resolving sore boils, and it is generally used externally by washing with its decocted water, spreading or applying on the affected areas after being grinded or smashed.

干檀香多生长于山坡灌木丛和向阳山坡处，除了它的叶可以入药以外，它的根也是一味很好的草药，每逢秋冬季将其采挖、洗净、切片、晒干以后就可以入药。干檀香根味辛，微苦，性凉，具有祛风、除湿、活血、止痛的功效。

It mostly grows in the hillside bushes or on the sunny hillsides, in addition to its leaves, its root is also a good herb. Dig it in autumn and winter and use them as medicine after being washed clean, sliced and dried in the sun. It tastes pungent and slightly bitter with cold property and has the effects of dispelling wind evil, eliminating dampness, promoting blood circulation and relieving pain.

57. 络石藤（络石）

Trachelospermum jasminoides（Lindl.）Lem.

以前在山野溪旁才能见到的络石，现在被人们作为花卉引种到了城市，它是夹竹桃科络石属常绿木质藤本植物。络石的干燥带叶藤茎和叶都是中药，其中药名就叫络石藤。它在我国的南方大部分省区都有分布。

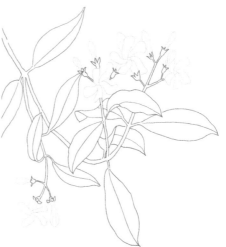

Trachelospermum jasminoides was used to be found on the hillsides or riversides, which is the evergreen woody vine plant of Apocynaceae and Trachelospermum, and it is now widely planted as flowers in cities. Its dried vine stem with leaves and leaves can be used as herbal medicine and its medicinal name is trachelospermum jasminoides, which is distributed in most of the Southern provinces of China.

其味苦，微寒，归心、肝、肾经，具有祛风通络、凉血消肿的功效，主治风湿热痹，喉痹，痈肿，跌扑损伤等病症。

It tastes bitter with minor cold property and belongs to heart, liver and kidney meridian. It has the effects of expelling wind and dredging meridian, cooling blood and removing swelling, and it can be used to treat rheumatic fever, pharyngitis, abscess and traumatic injuries.

58. 蓝莓（笃斯越桔） *Vaccinium uliginosum* L.

　　蓝莓是杜鹃花科越橘属植物笃斯越桔 Vaccinium uligino-sum L 的成熟新鲜果实；主要分布在中国主要分布于大兴安岭和小兴安岭林区。蓝莓（lanmei）的中药名叫越橘，《中华食疗本草》记载：其入药部位是叶和果实。其性凉，味甘、酸，归心、大肠经，具有降低胆固醇、增强心脏功能、防癌的功效，主治心脏功能不佳，心脏病等心脏疾患。

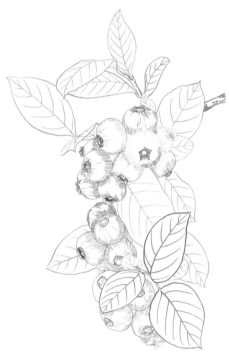

Blueberries are the ripe and fresh fruits of the Vaccinium uliginousm L. of Huckleberry of rhododendron family, which is mainly distributed in the forests of Greater Hinggan Mountains and Lesser Hinggan Mountains. It was recorded in *Chinese Diet Herbal Medinice* that its leaves and fruits can be used as herbal medicine, and it tastes sweet and sour with cold property, belongs to heart and large intestine meridian, it has the effects of lowering cholesterol, enhancing heart function and cancer prevention, it is mainly used to treat poor heart function and relevant heart diseases.

59. 金丝梅
Hypericum patulum Thunb.

金丝梅，为藤黄科金丝桃属植物。分布于江苏、浙江、安徽、福建、江西、湖北、湖南、广西、四川、云南等地。中药名亦称金丝梅，全株入药。其味苦，性寒，具有清热利尿、疏肝活络的功效，主治热淋、肝炎、感冒、扁桃体炎、疝气偏坠、筋骨疼痛、跌打损伤等病症。

Hypericum patulum Thunb. is the plant of Garcinia and Hypericum and distributes in Jiangsu, Zhejiang, Anhui, Fujian, Jiangxi, Hubei, Hunan, Guangxi, Sichuan and Yunnan. Its whole plant can be used as herbal medicine and its medicinal name is hypericum patulum. It tastes bitter with cold property and has the effects of clearing heat and inducing urine, soothing the liver and activating collaterals. It can be used to treat heat strangury, hepatitis, cold, amygdalitis, hernia, muscles and bones pain, traumatic injuries.

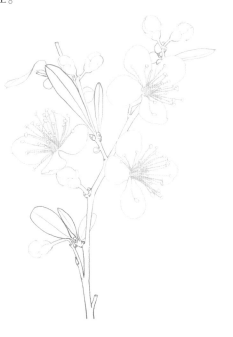

60. 白草莓（黄毛草莓）
Fragaria nilgerrensis Schltdl. ex. J. Gay

在山坡、草地、路旁、沟边，我们经常可以见到一种野果，它就是蔷薇科草莓属的多年生草本植物：黄毛草莓。

The wild fruits growing on the hillsides, meadows, roadsides and ditches are the fruits of perennial herb of Rosaceae and Fragaria of Fragaria nilgerrensis Schlecht. ex Gay.

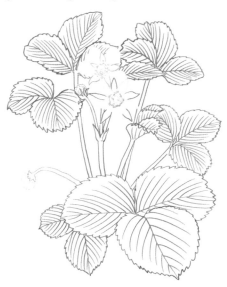

成熟的黄毛草莓的果实，是口感非常好的野果，它也曾是很多山村百姓童年的零食。黄毛草莓也是我们身边的一味草药，其中药名叫白草莓 Bai cao mei。其味甘、苦，性凉，具有清肺止咳、解毒消肿的功效，主治肺热咳喘、百日咳、口舌生疮、痢疾、淋证、疮疡肿痛、烫伤、毒蛇咬伤、骨折损伤等病症。

The ripe fruits of fragaria nilgerrensis schlecht are delicious wild fruits, which were once snacks for many people in mountain villages during their childnood. It is also a kind of herbal medicine around us and its medicinal name is Baicaomei it tastes sweet and bitter with cold property and it has the effects of removing heat from the lung to relieve cough, resolving toxin and dispersing swelling. It can be used to treat cough and panting due to lung heat, pertussis, mouth sores, dysentery, diarrhea, stranguria, sore boils, burns, venomous snake bites, fracture and traumatic injuries.

61. 万寿竹

Disporum cantoniense（Lour.）Merr

万寿竹是百合科万寿竹属的植物，在我国南方的大部分省区都有分布，在部分北方省区也有分布。万寿竹入药后有很多名字，在《中药大词典》和《中华本草》当中，把它叫作竹叶参；在《云南中草药》当中，把它叫作白根药、小竹根、倒竹散和老虎姜；而在《陕西中草药》当中，则把它叫作白龙须、竹叶七；在《贵州药植目录》当中，又把它叫作竹节参和石竹根。

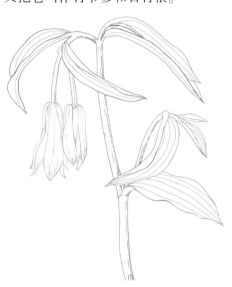

Disporum cantoniense is the plant of liliaceae and Disporum, which is distributed in most provinces in the Southern China and some Northern provinces. It owns several names, it is called Zhuyeshen in *Dictionary of Chinese Materia Medica* and *Chinese Herbal Medicine*, Baigenyao, Xiaozhugen, Daozhusan and Laohujiang in *Yunnan Chinese Herbal Medicine*, Bailongxu, Zhuyeqi in Shaanxi Chinese Herbal Medicine and Zhujieshen and Shizhugen in *Guizhou Medicine and Plant Catalog.*

万寿竹的根或根茎是入药部位，味苦、辛，性凉，归肝、肾经，具有祛风湿、舒筋活血、清热祛痰止咳之功效，用于风湿痹证、关节腰腿疼痛、跌打损伤、骨折、虚劳、骨蒸潮热、肺痨咯血、肺热咳嗽、烫火伤。

Its roots or stems can be used as herbal medicine and they taste bitter and pungent with cold property, belong to liver and kidney meridian. It has the effects of eliminating dampness, relaxing muscles and promoting blood circulation, clearing heat and expelling phlegm to relieve cough. It can be used to treat rheumatism syndrome, low back and leg pain, traumatic injuries, fractures, consumptive disease, hectic fever, pulmonary tuberculosis hemoptysis, lung heat cough, burns and scalds.

62. 松花（马尾松）   *Pinus massoniana* Lamb

松花又叫松花粉、松粉，为松科植物马尾松、油松、赤松、黑松等的花粉。

Pinus massoniana Lamb is the pollen of the Pinaceae plant of Pinusmassoniana Lamb, Pinus tabulaeformis Carr., Pinusdensiflora Sieb. et Zucc. and Pinus thunbergii Parl, it is also called Songhuafen and Songfen.

作为中药，其中药名就叫松花，是我们身边常见的一味草药，我国第一部药典《唐本草》就记载了松花的药用价值。其味甘，性温，归肝、胃经，无毒，具有祛风、益气、收湿、止血之功效，常用于头痛眩晕、泄泻下痢、湿疹湿疮、创伤出血等病症。

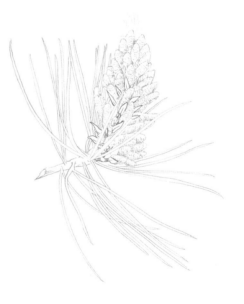

It is a common herbal medicine around us and its medicinal name is pinus massoniana lamb. Its medicinal value was illustrated in the first pharmacopoeia *Tang Materia Medica* that it is nontoxic and tastes sweet with warm property, belongs to liver and stomach meridian, and it has the effects of dispersing wind evil, tonifying Qi, removing dampness and stopping bleeding, it is often used to treat headache and dizziness, diarrhea, eczema and traumatic bleeding.

63. 牛至

Origanum vulgare L.

摘下这种植物的枝叶，揉搓以后可以散发出一股强烈的芳香气味，它就是唇形科牛至属植物牛至。云南人也把它叫作小叶薄荷、满坡香、土香薷和香草。在欧洲，人们是把它当做香料来食用的，而在我国它是一味很好的中药。

The leaves of this plant will give off a strong aromatic odor when rub them, which is the plant of Labiatae and Origanum. Yunnan people also call it Xiaoyebohe, Manpoxiang, Tuxiangru and Xiangcao. People take it as a spice in Europe, while it is a good medicinal herb in China.

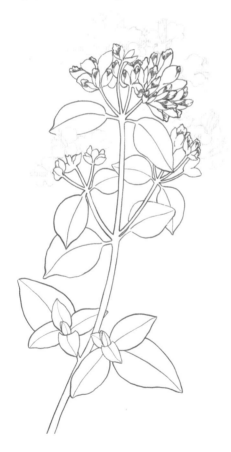

牛至在我国的分布很广，在云南等长江以南的大部分省区和部分北方省区都有分布。作为药用植物，其中药名就叫牛至，全草入药。其味辛、微苦，性凉，具有解表、理气、清暑、利湿的功效，主治感冒发热、中暑、胸膈胀满、腹痛吐泻、痢疾、黄疸、水肿、带下、小儿疳积、麻疹、皮肤瘙痒、疮疡肿痛、跌打损伤等病症。

Niuzhi is widely distributed in China, such as Yunnan and most Southern provinces of the Yangtze River, and even some Northern provinces also have its distribution. Its whole plant can be used as herbal medicine, which tastes pungent and slightly bitter with cold property, and has the effects of relieving exterior syndrome, regulating Qi circulation, clearing summer-heat, eliminating damp-ness. It can be used to treat cold and fever, sunstroke, chest fullness and disten-tion, abdominal pain, vomiting and diarrhea, dysentery, jaundice, edema, leu-corrhea, infantile malnutrition, measles, skin itch, sore and swollen boils as well as traumatic injuries.

64. 大白杜鹃 *Rhododendron decorum* Franch.

进入五月中下旬的香格里拉，满山遍野的大树杜鹃已经凋零，没有了踪影，而这个时候的大白杜鹃则开的正盛，和高原的朵朵白云交相辉映。

Rhododendron decorum Franch. all over the mountains are withering and disappearing in Shangri-La during the mid to late May, while the Rhododendron decorum is in full blossom and reflecting with the white clouds of the plateau.

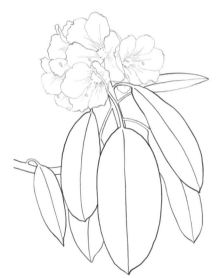

大白杜鹃分布于四川、贵州、云南、西藏，它的花朵美丽纯洁，具有很好的观赏价值，它还是我们身边的一味草药。作为药用植物，其中药名就叫大白杜鹃，其入药部位为杜鹃花科杜鹃花属植物大白花杜鹃的根、叶。其叶全年可采，而其根一般要到夏秋之际，采挖、洗净、切片、晒干以后就可以入药。其味辛，性平，归膀胱经，具有清利湿热、活血止痛的功效，主治白浊、带下、风湿疼痛、跌打损伤等病症。

Rhododendron decorum distributes in Sichuan, Guizhou, Yunnan and Xizang, its flowers are not only beautiful and pure with good ornamental value, but they are also the herbal medicine around us. Its roots and leaves can be used as herbal medicine and their medicinal name is Dabaidujuan Its leaves can be harvested all year round and its roots can be dug during summer and autumn, use them as medicine after being washed clean, sliced and dried in the sun. They taste pungent with mild property and belongs to bladder meridian, and they have the effects of eliminating dampness heat, promoting blood circulation to relieve pain. They can be used to treat gonorrhea, leucorrhea, rheumatic pain and traumatic injuries.

65. 长叶车前

Plantago lanceolata L.

　　长叶车前和我们经常见到的车前草，长相完全不一样，它的叶子细长细长的，花也长得很特别，所以把它叫作长叶车前，也把它叫作窄叶车前。

　　Plantago lanceolata L. is completely different from plantain in shape that we often see, which has long and thin leaves with unique flowers, so it is called Changyecheqian(Plantago lanceolata) , or Zhaiyecheqian.

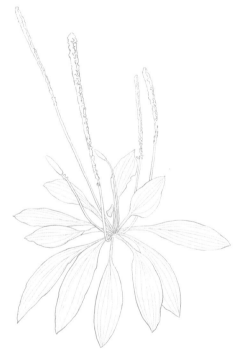

　　这种车前草科车前草属的多年生草本植物，分布于云南、江苏、浙江、江西、辽宁、甘肃、新疆、山东等地。

　　It is the perennial herb of Plantaginaceae and Plantago and distributes in Yunnan, Jiangsu, Zhejiang, Jiangxi, Liaoning, Gansu, Xinjiang and Shandong.

　　虽然它的功效和作用与我们经常说的车前草非常相似，但是在常见的中药书中找不到它的记载，在《中国饲用植物志》第六卷电子版当中却找到了相关内容。作为药用植物，其中药名就叫长叶车前。它全草可以入药，性寒，味甘，具有清热、明目、利尿、止泻、降血压、镇咳、祛痰等功效，主治泌尿系感染、高血压、结石、肾炎水肿、小便不利、肠炎、细菌性痢疾、急性黄疸型肝炎、支气管炎等病症。

　　Although its efficacy and usage are very similar to that of plantain, there is no record of it in common Chinese medicine books. While in Volume 6 Electronic edition of *Forage Flora of China* records that its whole plants can be used as medicine and its medicinal name is Changyecheqian and it tastes sweet with cold property. It has the effects of clearing heat, improving eyesight, inducing urine, relieving diarrhea, reducing blood pressure, relieving cough and eliminating phlegm. It can be used to treat urinary infection, hypertension, calculus, nephritic edema, inhibited urination, enteritis, bacillary dysentery, acute icteric hepatitis and bronchitis.

66. 吴茱萸

Tetradium ruticarpum (A. Juss.) T. G. Hartley

吴茱萸是芸香科吴茱萸属的植物，广泛分布于我国南方各省区和陕西、甘肃等部分北方省区。嫩果经泡制晾干后即是传统中药吴茱萸植物来源之一，简称吴萸。其味辛、苦，性热，有小毒，归肝、脾、胃、肾经，具有散寒止痛、降逆止呕、助阳止泻的功效，主治寒凝疼痛、胃寒呕吐、虚寒泄泻等病症。

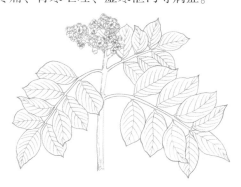

Tetradium ruticarpum(A. Juss.) T. G. Hartley is the plant of Rutaceae and Evodia Forst, which is widely distributed in Southern provinces of China as well as in Shaanxi and Gansu provinces. Its young fruits can be used as medicine after being soaked and dried in the shade, and its called Wuyu for short. It has minor toxicity and tastes pungent and bitter with hot property, belongs to liver, spleen, stomach and kidney meridian, and it has the effects of expelling cold to relieve pain, relieving nausea, supplying Yang to relieve diarrhea. It can be used to treat cold stagnation pain, vomiting due to stomach cold, diarrhea caused by deficiency and cold.

67. 龙眼

Dimocarpus longan Lour.

龙眼，无患子科龙眼属常绿乔木。这种水果在两广和滇南非常常见，又叫桂圆。作为药用植物，其中药名就叫龙眼，入药部位为龙眼的根、叶、假种皮（龙眼肉）及种子（龙眼核）。

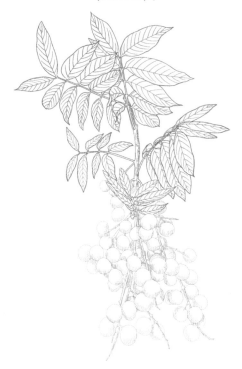

Dimocarpus longan Lour. is the evergreen arbor of Sapindaceae and Dimocarpus, which is commonly seen in Guangxi, Guangdong and Southern Yunnan, and it is also called longan. Its roots, leaves, longan flesh and seeds can be used as herbal medicine and their medicinal name is longan.

龙眼分布于云南、福建、台湾、广西、广东、四川、贵州等省区。龙眼的味道十分甜美，是一味好吃的中药。据《中药大词典》、《中华本草》和《全国中草药汇编》介绍：其根、叶味微苦，性平；假种皮味甘，性平；种子味微苦、涩，性平。

Longyan. tastes sweet and it is a delicious Chinese medicine, mainly distributes in Yunnan, Fujian, Taiwan, Guangxi, Guangdong, Sichuan and Guizhou. According to *Dictionary of Chinese Materia Medica*, *Chinese Herbal Medicine* and *National Compilation of Chinese Herbal Medicine*, its roots and leaves taste slightly bitter with mild property, its longan flesh tastes sweet with mild property and its longan seeds taste slightly bitter and astringent with mild property.

龙眼的功效主要有：根利湿，通络，主治乳糜尿、白带、风湿关节痛。叶清热解毒、解表利湿，可预防流行性感冒，治疗流行性脑脊髓膜炎、感冒、肠炎，外用治阴囊湿疹。假种皮补心脾、养血安神，主治病后体虚、神经衰弱、健忘、心悸、失眠。种子止血、止痛，主治胃痛、烧烫伤、刀伤出血、疝气痛，外用治外伤出血。

Its roots have the effects of eliminating dampness and dredging collaterals, and they can be used to treat chyluria, leucorrhea, rheumatic joint pain. Its leaves have the effects of clearing heat and removing toxicity, relieving exterior syndrome and eliminating dampness, and they can be used to prevent influenza, epidemic cerebrospinal meningitis, cold, enteritis and external treatment for scrotal eczema. Its longan flesh can tonify heart and spleen, nourish blood and calm the nerves, and it can be used to treat weakness after illness, neurasthenia, forgetfulness, palpitation and insomnia. Its longan seeds can stop bleeding and relieve pain, and they can be used to treat stomachache, burns and scalds, knife wound bleeding, colic pain and external treatment for traumatic bleeding.

68. 苍耳

Xanthium sibiricum L.

在云南的山坡、草地、路旁、沟边，到处可以见到这种长满小刺球的植物，小孩子们常把小刺球摘下来，作为男孩子相互攻击打闹的玩具。这就是菊科苍耳属一年生草本植物苍耳的成熟带总苞的果实。

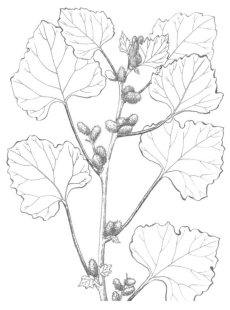

The plant with small prickly balls can be seen everywhere on the slopes, grasslands, roadsides and ditches in Yunnan, children often pick the little thorn balls off as a toy for attacking and fighting each other, which are the ripe fruits with involucre of annual herb of Compositae and Xanthium L.

苍耳分布于全国各地，每逢深秋，当苍耳由绿转黄、茎叶也枯萎的时候，就可以采摘了，洗净晒干，炒至微黄就可以入药。作为药用植物，其中药名就叫苍耳子，其味辛、苦，性温，有毒，归肺经，具有发散风寒、通鼻窍、祛风湿、止痛的功效，主治风寒感冒、鼻渊、风湿痹痛、风疹瘙痒、疥癣麻风等病症。

It distributes throughout China and its fruits can be harvested when they are turning to yellow from green and its stems and leaves are withering in late autumn, and they can be used as medicine after being washed clean and fried to light yellow. Its medicinal name is Cangerzi and it is toxic and tastes pungent and bitter with warm property, belongs to lung meridian. It has the effects of dispersing wind cold, clearing the nasal passage, eliminating rheumatism and relieving pain. It can be used to treat wind-cold, nasosinusitis, rheumatic arthralgia, rubella pruritus, scabies and leprosy.

69. 肿节风（草珊瑚）

Sarcandra glabra（Thunb.）Nakai

肿节风作为一种中药，它有很多名字，又叫草珊瑚、九节风、接骨木、九节茶、接骨丹、接骨草、山牛膝，还有人把它叫作铜角威灵仙，是金粟兰科草珊瑚属植物草珊瑚的干燥全株。

Zhongjiefeng is also called Caoshanhu, Jiujiefeng, Jiegumu, Jiujiecha, Jiegudan, Jiegucao, Shanniuxi or Tongjiaoweilingxian, which is the dried plant of Chloranthaceae and Sarcandra.

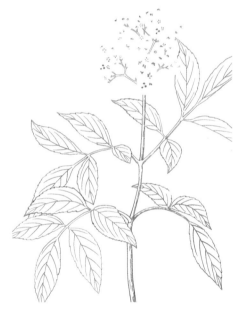

草珊瑚在我国南方的大部分省市都有分布，其味辛、苦，性平，归肝、大肠经。全草或根是入药部位，具有祛风活血、清热解毒的功效，主治风湿痹痛、肢体麻木、跌打损伤、骨折、痛经、瘀滞腹痛、流感、肺炎、急性阑尾炎、急性胃肠炎、菌痢、脓肿等病症。

It is distributed in most provinces and cities in southern China and it tastes pungent and bitter with mild property, belongs to liver and large intestine meridian. Its whole plant or roots can be used as herbal medicine and they have the effects of expelling wind and promoting blood circulation, clearing heat and removing toxicity. It can be used to treat rheumatic arthralgia, limb numbness, traumatic injuries, fractures, dysmenorrhea, abdominal pain due to stasis after delivery, flu, pneumonia, acute appendicitis, acute gastroenteritis, dysentery and abscess.

70. 鸡脚刺（豪猪刺） *Berberis julianae* Schneid

小檗科小檗属植物豪猪刺，外形与三颗针很像，但是两者是同科同属不同种。

Berberis julianae Schneid is the plant of berberis silva-taroucana Schneid family and genus, its shape resembles barberry and belong to the same family and genus but in different species.

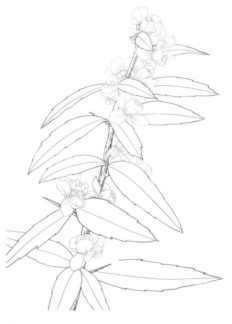

中药三颗针是小檗科小檗属细叶小檗或刺黑珠的根、茎或树皮，而鸡脚刺则是小檗科小檗属豪猪刺的根或茎。

Sankezhen is the root, stem or bark of Berberis poiretii schneid or acanthophora spinosa that belongs to berberis silva-taroucana Schneid family and genus, while Jijiaoci is the root or stem of Berberis julianae Schneid family and genus that its thorn has been removed.

在云南，也有人把鸡脚刺叫作三颗针，但无论是三颗针还是鸡脚刺，它们所含的主要成分都是小檗碱。

People in Yunnan also call it as barberry, but whether it is Jijiaoci or barberry, they contain the main component of berberine.

鸡脚刺又叫豪猪刺、三个针、九铃小檗，这种常绿灌木主要分布在江西、湖北、湖南、四川、云南、陕西，它主要生长于海拔1100—1700米的向阳杂林当中，每逢秋季都可以采收，将其洗净、切片、晒干以后就可以入药。

Jijiaoci is also called Haozhuci, Sangezhen, Jiulingxiaopi, this evergreen shrub mainly distributes in Jiangxi, Hubei, Hunan, Sichuan, Yunnan and Shannxi, it mainly grows in sunlit forest at elevations of 1, 100 m to 1, 700 m. It can be harvested every autumn and used as medicine after being washed, sliced and dried.

其味苦，性寒，无毒，具有清热解毒的功效，主治泄泻、痢疾、湿热黄疸、眼赤肿痛、疮毒。

It tastes bitter with cold property and nontoxic, and it has the effects of clearing heat and detoxifying. It can be used to treat diarrhea, dysentery, dampness-heat jaundice, red and sore eyes, sore toxin.

71. 白簕
Eleutherococcus trifoliatus（L.）S. Y. Hu

这种攀岩灌木叫白簕，为五加科植物白簕的全株都可以入药。白簕的中药名叫三加，也叫它白刺根、三叶五加、刺三加、苦刺根、簕勾菜。

Eleutherococcus trifoliatus（L.）S. Y. Hu is a kind of rock-climbing shrub and is the plant of Araliaceae, it whole plant Its medicinal name is called Sanjia, Baicigen, Sanyewujia, Cisanjia, Kucigen or Legoucai.

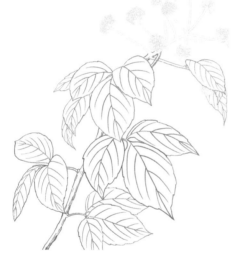

白簕主要分布于我国中南部，云南宾川等地多见。它多生长于河边、村旁山坡或者是陵园灌木丛中，它的根叶和全株一年四季都可以采收，将其晒干就可以入药，鲜品也可以使用。

Baile is mainly distributed in Middle of South, and it is commonly seen in Binchuan county of Yunnan province. It mostly grows in the riversides, the hillsides next to the village or in the bushes of the cemetery, its roots and leaves as well as the whole plant can be harvested all year round, and it can be used as medicine after being dried in the sun or use its fresh leaves or roots directly.

其味苦、涩，性凉，具有清热解毒、祛风除湿、散瘀止痛的功效，常用于黄疸、肠炎、胃痛、风湿性关节炎、腰腿痛，外用治跌打损伤、疮疖肿毒、湿疹。

Baile tastes bitter and astringent with cold property, it has the effects of clearing heat and removing toxicity, dispelling wind and eliminating dampness, relieving pain by dissipating stasis. It is often used for treating jaundice, enteritis, stomach pain, rheumatoid arthritis, lumbar and leg pain, and traumatic injuries, sore and furuncle, eczema for external use.

72. 接骨木 *Sambucus williamsii* Hance

接骨木是忍冬科接骨木属的植物，它的茎枝也是可以拿来入药的。接骨木在云南及我国的大部分地区都有分布，它多生长于林下、灌木或者平原路旁。其中药名也叫接骨木，干燥带叶茎入药每逢5—7月份可以采收，将其洗净、晒干以后就可以入药，鲜品也可以入药。

Sambucus williamsii Hance is the plant of honeysuckle and sambucus williamsii hance family, its stems and

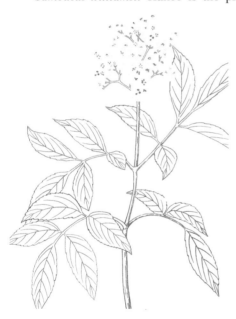

branches can be used as herbal medicine. It is widely distributed in Yunan and most of China and mainly grows in the bushes or plain roadsides. Its medicinal name is Jiegumu and its dried stems with leaves can be used as herbal medic in It can be collected May to July, and its fresh stems and branches can be used as herbal medicine directly or use them after being washed clean and dried in the sun.

其味甘、苦，性平，归肝经，具有祛风利湿、活血止血的功效，主治风湿痹痛、痛风、大骨节病、急慢性肾炎、风疹、跌打损伤、骨折肿痛、外伤出血。

It tastes sweet and bitter with mild property, belongs to liver meridian. It has the effects of dispelling wind and removing dampness, and it is mainly used to treat rheumatic arthralgia, gout, kaschin-beck disease, acute and chronic nephritis, urticaria, traumatic injuries, swelling and pain of fractures, traumatic bleeding.

73. 过山青　　*Reinwardtia indica* Dumort.

　　过山青是一种直立小灌木，为亚麻科植物石海椒的嫩枝叶，分布于云南、湖北、广西、四川、贵州等地。它主要生长于路边，山坡，或者沟边的草丛中。

　　Reinwardtia indica Dumort. is a kind of upright shrub, it is the tender branches and leaves of linaceae family of Reinwardtia indica Dumort. R. trigyna(Roxb.) Planch. It is distributed in Yunnan, Hubei, Guangxi, Sichuan and Guizhou provinces and mainly grows in roadside slopes or ditch grass clusters.

　　其中药名就叫过山青，其味甘，性寒，具有清热利尿的功效，常用于小便不利、肾炎、黄疸型肝炎。

　　Its medicinal name is Guoshanqing and it tastes sweet with cold property and has the effects of clearing heat and diuretic, and it is mainly used to treat dysuria, nephritis and icteric hepatitis.

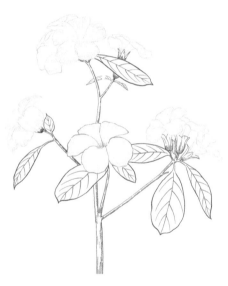

74. 水(杨)柳 *Homonoia riparia* Lour.

水杨柳又叫水柳，它是大戟科植物。这种矮小灌木多生长于云南东南部至西南部，广东、广西、台湾，它多生长于河旁沙地中，溪边石缝中以及山坡灌木丛中。其皮、叶、根入药，根全年都可以采挖，将其采挖洗净、切片晒干以后就可以入药。

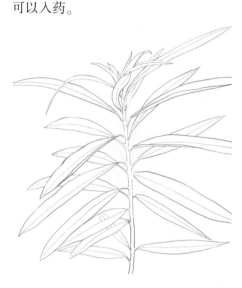

Homonoia riparia Lour. is also called Shuiliu, it is the plant of Euphorbiaceae of Homonoia riparia Lour. It is a short and small shrub and mainly distributes in Southeast and Southwest of Yunnan province, Guangdong, Guangxi and Taiwan, and it mostly grows in the sand beside the river, the crevices beside the stream and in the bushes on the hillside. Its medicinal name is Shuiliu and it barks, leaves. and roots can be used as horbal medicine. It can be harvested all year round and it can be used as herbal medicine after being washed clean, sliced and dried in the sun.

其味苦，性寒；归肝、胆、膀胱经，具有清热、利胆、利尿、解毒的功效，主治急慢性肝炎、胆囊炎、胆结石、膀胱结石、淋病、梅毒、痔疮、跌打损伤、烫伤。

It tastes bitter with cold property and belongs to liver, gallbladder and urinary bladder meridian. It has the effects of clearing heat, increasing choleresis and diuresis as well as detoxification, and it is mainly used to treat acute and chronic hepatitis, cholecystitis, gallstones, bladder stones, gonorrhea, syphilis, hemorrhoids, traumatic injuries and scald.

75. 白及

Bletilla striata (Thunb. ex A. Murray) Rchb. f.

白及为兰科白及属植物。分布于云南、陕西南部、甘肃东南部等地区常绿阔叶林下，树林或针叶林下、路边草丛或岩石缝中。

Bletilla striata(Thunb. ex A. Murray) Rchb. f. is the plant orchid family of Bletillastriata(Thunb.) Reichb. f. . It is mostly distributed in Yunnan, South of Shannxi, Southeast of Gansu, and grows in evergreen broad-leaved forest, taiga forest, roadside bushes or rock crevice.

块茎入药，叫白及，其味苦、甘、涩，性微寒，归肺、胃、肝经，具有收敛止血、消肿生肌的功效，主治出血证，痈肿疮疡，手足皲裂，水火烫伤。

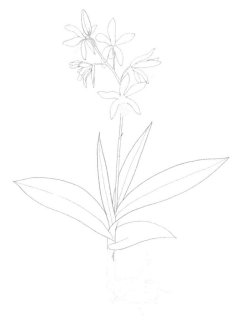

Its medicinal name is Baiji and it paeonia lactiflora. Pall is the plant of the genus Paeonia of Buttercup family. It has beautiful flowers, and its roots are @ herbal medicine commonly used. tastes bitter, sweet and astringent with minor cold, belongs to lung, stomach and liver meridian. It has the effects of astringing to stop bleeding, removing detumescence and promoting granulation. It is mainly used to treat hemorrhagic syndrome, sores and carbuncles, chapped hands and feet, burn from hot liquid or fire.

76. 白芍（芍药）

Paeonia lactiflora Pall.

芍药为毛茛科芍药属植物。芍药不仅具有美丽的花朵，其根也是一味我们常用的中药。芍药的生长期一般为 2 到 3 年，其根每逢夏秋都可以采挖，采挖后除去外皮，加工以后就成白芍，具有养血敛阴、柔肝止痛、平抑肝阳的功效。

Paeonia lactiflora Pall. is not only a kind of beautiful flower, but also a common herbal medicine, its roots used as medicinal herbs are the plant of Ranunculaceae family of Paeonia lactiflora Pall. Its growth period is generally 2 to 3 years and its roots can be harvested every summer and autumn, then remove its skin to make it into Baishao. It has the effects of nourishing blood and restraining Yin, soothing liver and relieving pain and calming liver Yang.

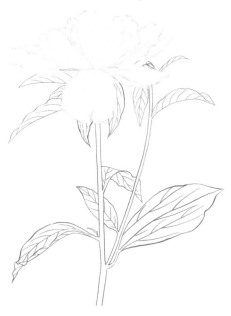

芍药主要分布于云南大理北部、云南大部分地区、西藏、四川、广西、湖南等地。白芍味苦、酸，性微寒，归肝、脾经，主治肝血亏虚、月经不调、肝脾不和、胸胁脘腹疼痛、四肢挛急疼痛、肝阳上亢、头痛眩晕等。

Paeonia lactiflora Pall. is manily distributed in the North of Dali, most areas of Yunnan, Xizang, Sichuan, Guangxi and Hunan. Its medicinal name is Baishao and it tastes bitter and sour with minor cold property, belongs to liver and spleen meridian. It is mainly used to treat liver blood depletion, irregular menstruation, disharmony between liver and spleen, chest, hypochondriac duct and abdomen pain, acute clonic pain in the extremities, hyperactivity of liver-Yang, headache and dizziness.

77. 朱唇

Salvia coccinea Buc'hoz ex Etl.

朱唇，为唇形科鼠尾草属一年生或者多年生草本植物。这种植物如今常常在城市的绿化带、小区花园里见到，云南人也叫它金鱼花、三叶青、香茶菜、小红花和丹参。朱唇也是可以入药的，入药部分为全草。在《全国中草药汇编》和《中药大词典》里都有详细的记载。

Salvia coccinea Buc'hoz ex Etl. is an annual or perennial herb of Salvia labiaceae, it can be found in urban green belts and community gardens. It is also called Jinyuhua, Sanyeqing, Xiangchacai, Xiaohonghua and Danshen by Yunnan people, its whole plant can be used as medicine and its usage was recorded in detail in *National Compilation of Chinese Herbal Medicine* and *Dictionary of Chinese Herbal Medicine*.

它原产于美洲，在云南及全国都有栽种，常作为观赏植物。它入药也叫朱唇，每逢 6—9 月份可以采收，将其洗净晒干以后就可以入药。其味辛、微苦、涩，性凉，具有凉血止血、清热利湿的功效，用于血崩、高热、腹痛不适等病症的治疗。

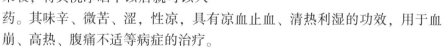

It is native to America, and cultivated in Yunnan and all over China and often regarded as an ornamental plant. It can be harvested from June to September every year and it can be used as herbal medicine after being washed cleanly and dried in the sun. Its medicinal name is Zhuchun and it tastes pungent, slightly bitter and astringent with cold property, and it has the effects of cooling blood to stop bleeding, clearing heat and draining dampness. It is mainly used for treating metrorrhagia, high fever and abdominal pain.

78. 滇黄精

Polygonatum kingianum Collett & Hemsl

被纳入中药使用的黄精一共有三种，植物为百合科黄精属植物黄精、多花黄精和滇黄精。其用药部分皆为干燥根茎。

Huangjing is a name of Chinese materia medica and there are three kinds plant of Polygonatum sibiricum Red. , Polygonatum cyrtonema Hua and Polygonatum kingianum Coll. et Hemsl. that can be used as herbal medicine. its dried roots and stems can be used ac herbal medicine

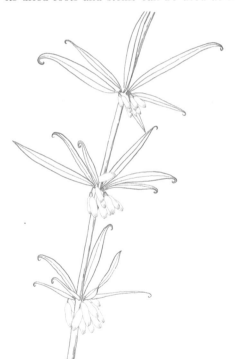

其中，滇黄精主要分布在西南地区和广西，它多生长于林下、灌木丛中和阴湿草坡上，每年9—10月份是采收的季节，将其采收、洗净、切片，晒干以后就可以入药。其味甘，性平，归脾、肺、肾经，具有养阴润肺、补脾益气、滋肾填精的功效，主治阴虚劳嗽、肺燥咳嗽、脾虚乏力、食少口干、消渴、肾亏腰膝酸软、阳痿遗精、耳鸣目暗、须发早白、体虚羸瘦、风癞癣疾等病症。

Polygonatum kingianum Colloet Hemsl, is mainly distributed in Southwest China and Guangxi. and mostly grows in the bushes and wet grassy slopes. It can be harvested from September to October every year and it can be used as herbal medicine after being washed clean, sliced and dried in the sun. It tastes sweet with mild property and belongs to spleen, lung and kidney meridian, and it has the effects of nourishing Yin and moistening lung, invigorating spleen and replenishing Qi, nourishing kidney and replenishing essence. It is mainly used to treat cough due to Yin deficiency, lung dryness cough, weakness due to spleen deficiency, poor appetite and dry mouth, diabetes, soreness and weakness of waist and knees caused by kidney deficiency, impotence and spermatogenesis, tinnitus and dim eyesight, premature graying of hair, thin and weak body, leprosy and tinea.

79. 小报春花（小报春） *Primula forbesii* Franch.

进入春季，云南满山遍野的报春花令人陶醉。不仅花市上有报春花出售，药材市场上也能见到它的身影。小报春为报春花科报春花属植物，它也是我们身边的一味草药，入药部分全草。该植物分布于云南的鹤庆、邓川、洱源、昆明、宜良、澄江、蒙自等地。

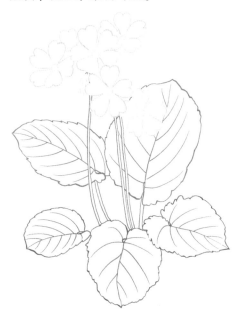

People are intoxicated by the primroses all over the mountains in Yunnan during springtime. Not only are primroses sold in the flower market, but they can also be seen in the medicinal herbs market, Xiaobaochunhua is a kind of herbal medicine in our daily usage and its whole plant can be used as medicine. It mainly distributes in Heqing County, Dengchuan County, Eryuan County, Kunming City, Yiliang County, Chengjiang County and Mengzi County in Yunnan province.

其味辛、微甘，性凉，具有清热解毒、消肿止痛的功效，主治高热咳嗽、小儿肺炎、咽喉炎、口腔炎、扁桃腺炎、牙痛、急性结膜炎、肾炎、风湿关节痛、产后出血、红崩白带、外伤出血、跌打瘀血等病症。

It tastes pungent and slight sweet with cold property, and it has the effects of clearing heat and removing toxicity, relieving swelling and pain. It is mainly used to treat cough with high fever, infantile pneumonia, pharyngitis, stomatitis, tonsillitis, toothache, acute conjunctivitis, nephritis, rheumatic joint pain, postpartum hemorrhage, heavy bleeding during menstruation and leucorrhea, traumatic bleeding and blood stasis caused by traumatic injuries.

80. 五蕊寄生

Dendrophthoe pentandra（L.）Miq.

五蕊寄生，是一种桑寄生科五蕊寄生属寄生性灌木。分布于我国云南、广西、广东等地，在东南亚等地也有分布。五蕊寄生有多个名字，它又叫茶树寄生、木菠萝寄生、乌榄树寄生、黑榄树寄生、木微子寄生和芒果木寄生。作为一种中药，其中药名叫五蕊寄生，其入药部位为植物五蕊寄生的带叶茎枝。

Dendrophthoe pentandra（L.）Miq. is a parasitic shrub of loranthaceae and dendrophthoe, mainly distributes in Yunnan, Guangxi, Guangdong as well as in Southeast Asia. It has several names, such as tea tree parasitism, jackfruit parasitism, dark olive parasitism, black olive parasitism, Muweizi parasitism and mango wood parasitism. As a kind of herbal medicine, its medicinal name is Wurui Jisheng, and its stems and branches with leaves can be used as medicine.

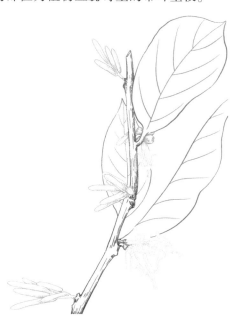

其味苦、甘，性平，入肝、肾、脾经，有祛风湿、补肝肾、止泻痢的功效，主治风湿痹痛、腰痛、腰膝酸软、腹泻、痢疾。

It tastes bitter and sweet with mild property, belongs to liver, kidney and spleen meridian. It has the effects of dispelling wind-damp, nourishing liver and kidney, relieving diarrhea and dysentery, and can be used to treat rheumatic arthralgia, backache, soreness and weakness of waist and knees, diarrhea and dysentery.

81. 南板蓝根（板蓝）   *Strobilanthes cusia*（Nees）kuntze

 中药南板蓝根为爵床科植物板蓝的干燥根和根茎，每年11—12 月份将其采挖，除去杂质，洗净，润透，切厚片，干燥后入药。该植物主要分布于云南、福建、四川、湖南、江西、贵州、广东、广西等地。

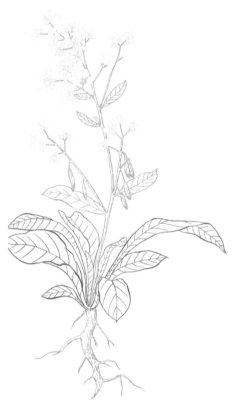

Nanbanlangen is a Chinese medicine name, its medicinal parts are the dried roots and stems of the euphorbia family of Radin Isatidis, it can be harvested from November and December every year and used as herbal medicine after removing the impurities and being washed clean, moistened thoroughly, sliced into thick pieces and dried. It distributes in places such as Yunnan, Fujian, Sichuan, Hunan, Jiangxi, Guizhou, Guangdong and Guangxi Zhuang Autonomous Region.

其味苦，性寒，入肝、胃经，具有清热解毒、避疫杀虫的功效，主治伤寒发斑、丹毒、瘟疫发颐及大头瘟等病症。

It tastes bitter with cold property, belongs to liver and stomach meridian, it has the effects of clearing heat and removing toxicity, preventing epidemic disease and killing insects. It is mainly used to treat typhoid fever spots, erysipelas, plague and infection with swollen head.

82. 野洋参(滇北球花报春)
Primula denticulata subsp. *sinodenticulata*

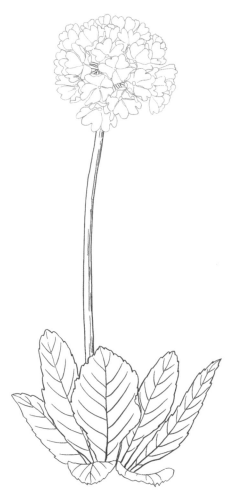

中药野洋参是报春花科报春花属植物滇北球花报春的根。它的中药名又叫报春花根，每逢夏季将其采收，洗净、晒干以后就可以入药，鲜品也可以使用。进入3月，滇西地区野外的山坡上，到处开满了这种淡紫色的小花，令人赏心悦目。它多生长于海拔1500米到3000米的山坡草地和灌木丛中，每年6—7月份，我们将其采挖、洗净、切片，晒干以后就可以入药。

Yeyangshen is the root of primulaceae and platymiscium plant of primula, its medicinal name is Sanyuehua and it can be used as herbal medicine after being harvested in summer, washed clean and dried in the sun, or use its fresh plants directly. There are full of tiny purple flowers all over the wild hillsides in Western Yunnan in March, which is pleasing to our eyes. It mostly grows in grass and shrubs at altitudes of 1500 to 3000 meters of hillside, it can be harvested from June to July every year and used as herbal medicine after being washed clean, sliced and dried in the sun.

其味甘、辛，性微温，归肺经，具有补虚、消疳、通乳的功效，用于虚劳咳嗽、病后体虚、小儿疳积、妇人气血不足之乳汁不下

119

等病症的治疗。

It tastes sweet and pungent with minor warm property, belongs to lung meridian, and it has the effects of tonifying deficiency, destroying parasites for curing malnutrition and promoting lactation. It is mainly used to treat cough due to deficiency and fatigue, weakness after disease, infantile malnutrition, stoppage of lactation caused by lack of Qi and blood.

83. 鸭嘴花　　*Justicia adhatoda* L.

鸭嘴花为爵床科鸭嘴花属植物。全株可入药，中药名也叫大驳骨、大驳骨萧、牛舌兰。它全年都可以采收，该植物分布于广东、广西、海南、澳门、香港、云南等地区。

The medicinal name of *Justicia adhatoda* L. is called Dabogu, which is the root and stem of acanthus family of Adhatoda vasi-caNees. Some people also call it Dabogu, Daboguxiao or Niushelan. It can be harvested all year round and it distributes in Guangdong, Guangxi, Hainan, Macao, Hongkong and Yunnan.

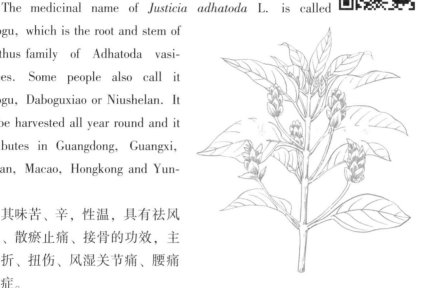

其味苦、辛，性温，具有祛风活血、散瘀止痛、接骨的功效，主治骨折、扭伤、风湿关节痛、腰痛等病症。

It tastes bitter and pungent with warm property, and it has the effects of dispelling wind and promoting blood circulation, eliminating stagnant blood to relieve pain and setting a broken bone. It is mainly used to treat fracture, sprain, rheumatic joint pain and lumbago.

84. 菩提树　　*Ficus religiosa* L.

　　菩提树，桑科榕属的常绿乔木。在云南的西双版纳、德宏等地，常常会看到很多佛寺里有郁郁葱葱的菩提树。其中还有很多非常有特色的树包塔、塔包树。菩提树蕴含着很多宗教、文化内涵，也有很多故事，它还是一味很好的中药，作为药用植物，其中药名叫菩提树，其入药部位为菩提树的树皮。

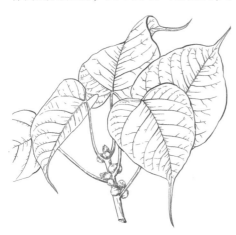

Ficus religiosa L. is an evergreen arbor of Moraceae and Ficus, we can often see a lot of lush bodhi trees in Buddhist temples in Xishuangbanna and Dehong in Yunnan, and there is also distinctive scene that a tower in a bodhi tree and a bodhi tree in a tower among them. Therefore, bodhi tree not only contains many religious, cultural connotations and many stories, but it is also a good herbal medicine, and its Chinese medicine name is called Putishu as a medicinal plant, and its bark can be used as herbal medicine.

　　其味苦，性寒，归肝经，具有止痛、固齿的功效，常用于牙痛、牙齿浮动。

It tastes bitter with cold property and belongs to liver meridian, it has the effects of relieving pain and strengthening teeth, and it is often used to theat toothache and teeth looseness.

85. 西南文殊兰　　*Crinum latifolium* L.

西南文殊兰是石蒜科文殊兰属植物，分布于云南、广西、四川、贵州等地。它的中药名就叫西南文殊兰，全草入药，全年都可以采收，将其洗净、切碎、晒干就可以备用，鲜品也可以使用。

Crinum latifolium L. is a plant of Amaryllidaceae and Crinum, and distributes in Yunnan, Guangxi, Sichuan and Guizhou. Its medicinal name is Xinan Wenshulan it can be harvested all year round and used as medicinal herb after being washed clean, sliced and dried in the sun, or use its fresh plants directly.

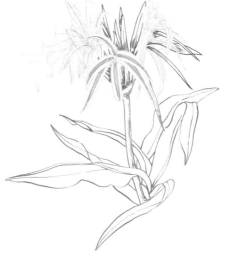

其味辛、苦，性凉，归肝、胃经，小毒，具有活血祛瘀、通络止痛、清热解毒的功效，用于跌打伤肿、骨折、关节痛、牙痛、恶疮肿毒、痔疮、带状疱疹、牛皮癣等病症。

It tastes bitter and pungent with cold property and mild toxicity, belongs to liver and stomach meridian. It has the effects of activating blood and removing stasis, regulating meridians to relieve pain, clearing heat and removing toxicity. It can be used to treat bruise injuries, fractures, joint pain, toothache, malignant sore and pyogenic infections, piles, herpes zoster and psoriasis.

86. 卷柏

Selaginella tamariscina（P. Beauv.）Spring

卷柏是多年生常绿草本植物，主要分布在云南、湖南、福建、四川、陕西、江西、浙江等地。作为药用植物，它的中药名就叫卷柏，是一味难得的中药，入药部分是卷柏科卷柏属的植物卷柏的干燥全草。每年春秋两季均可采收，将其洗净、晒干以后就可以备用。

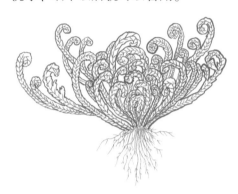

Selaginella tamariscina（P. Beauv.）Spring is a perennial evergreen herb, mainly distributed in Yunnan, Hunan, Fujian, Sichuan, Shaanxi, Jiangxi and Zhejiang provinces. As a medicinal plant, its medicinal name is Juanbai and its medicinal plants are Selaginella tamariscina（Beauv.）Spring or the whole dry herbs of Selaginella pulvinate（Hook. etGrev.）Maxim. It can be harvested in spring and autumn every year, and it can be used after being washed clean and dried in the sun.

其味辛，性平，归肝、心经，无毒，具有活血通经的功效，用于经闭痛经、癥瘕痞块、跌打损伤。卷柏炭还有化瘀止血的功效，用于吐血、崩漏、便血、脱肛等病症的治疗。

It tastes pungent with mild property and non-toxic, belongs to liver and heart meridian. It has the effects of promoting blood circulation and menstruation and it can be used to treat dysmenorrhea and amenorrhea, mass in the abdomen and traumatic injuries. In addition, sellodendron charcoal also has the effect of removing blood stasis and it can be used to treat hematemesis, uterine bleeding, hematochezia and rectocele.

87. 地黄

Rehmannia glutinosa（Gaert.）Libosch. ex Fisch. et Mey.

地黄是玄参科地黄属多年生草本植物。地黄在我国的分布很广，几乎从北到南，从东到西都有分布。地黄的入药部分是地黄的新鲜或干燥块根，一般分为鲜地黄、干地黄和熟地黄。我们把这种烘干以后的地黄根块叫作干地黄，每年10—11月份挖根、洗净、切片、烘炕以后就可以入药。地黄新鲜状态下的根茎就叫作鲜地黄，鲜地黄和干地黄的功效是有区别的，用黄酒拌匀、蒸透以后的地黄就叫作熟地黄。地黄除了根可以入药以外，它的花、果实以及叶也是可以拿来做药的，其中药名分别叫地黄花、地黄石和地黄叶。

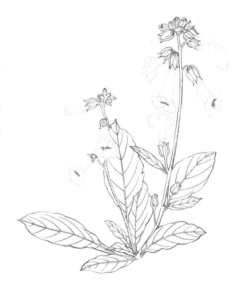

Rehmannia glutinosa (Gaert.) Libosch. ex Fisch. et Mey. is a perennial herb of Rehmannia glutinosa (Gaert.) Libosch. ex Fisch. et Mey., and distributes widely in China. Its fresh or dried roots can be used as medicinal herbs, and it is generally divided into fresh Rehmannia, dry Rehmannia and cooked Rehmannia. The dried root of Rehmannia is called dry Rehmannia, it can be harvested from October to November and used as medicine after being washed clean, sliced and dried by heating. The fresh root of Rehmannia is called fresh Rehmannia, and its effect is different from dried Rehmannia. While the cooked Rehmannia is mixed with rice wine evenly and steamed. In addition to its roots, its flowers, fruits and leaves can also be used as medicine, which are called Rehmannia flower, Rehmannia stone and Rehmannia leaf respectively.

干地黄：味甘，性寒。熟地黄：味甘，性微温，无毒。鲜地黄具有清热生津、凉血、止血的功效。干地黄具有清热凉血、养阴生津的功效。熟地黄具有补血滋阴、益精填髓的功效。

Dried Rehmannia tastes sweet with cold property, cooked Rehmannia tastes sweet with mild warm property and non-toxicity, fresh Rehmannia has the effects of removing heat and promoting salivation, cooling blood and stopping bleeding, dried Rehmannia can clear heat and cool blood, nourish Yin and generate body fluid, while cooked Rehmannia has the effects of replenishing blood and nourishing Yin, generating essence and supplementing marrow.

88. 老鼠簕

Acanthus ilicifolius L.

老鼠簕，是爵床科老鼠簕属的直立灌木植物。由于这种常绿有刺灌木浑身长满了荆棘，连老鼠都很难靠近，所以把它叫作老鼠簕，也有人叫它老鼠怕。老鼠簕分布于广东、海南、广西等地。它的根和枝叶是可以拿来做药的，中药名也叫老鼠簕。全年都可以采收，将其洗净、切断、晒干以后就可以备用。

It is an upright shrub of Acanthus family and ilicifolius L. genes, this evergreen thorny shrub is covered with thorns, even rats are difficult to get close to it, so it is called Acanthus ilicifolius L. or Laoshupa. It distributes in Guangdong, Hainan and Guangxi. its roots and leaves can be used as herbal medicine and its medicinal name is called Laoshule. It can be harvested all year round and used as medicine after being washed clean, cut and dried in the sun.

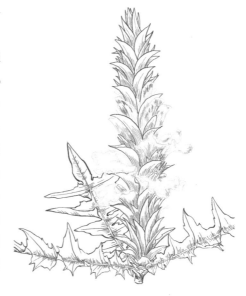

其味微苦，性凉，归肝、肺经，具有清热解毒、散瘀止痛、化痰利湿的功效，常用于疟腮、瘰疬、肝脾肿大、胃痛、腰肌劳损、痰热咳喘、黄疸、白浊等病症的治疗。

It tastes slightly bitter with cold property, belongs to liver and lung meridian. It has the effects of clearing heat and removing toxicity, relieving pain by dissipating blood stasis, resolving phlegm and eliminating dampness. It is commonly used to treat mumps, crewels, Hepatosplenomegaly, stomachache, strain of lumbar muscles, phlegm-heat cough and panting, jaundice and gonorrhea.

89. 柳叶栒子   *Cotoneaster salicifolius* Franch.

柳叶栒子为蔷薇科栒子属半常绿或常绿灌木，分布于西南及湖北、湖南等地。柳叶荀子作为盆栽，很受人们的欢迎，它还是一味中药，其中药名叫柳叶栒子，入药部位为植物全株。

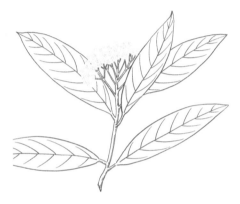

It is a semi-evergreen or evergreen shrub of Rosaceae and cotoneaster, distributes in Southwest China, Hubei and Hunan provinces. It is very popular as a potted plant and its whole plant can be used as medicinal herb and called Liuye Xun-zi.

其味苦，性凉，归肺、大肠、小肠经，无毒，具有清热祛风、止血利尿的功效，常用于干咳失音、湿热发黄、肠风下血、小便短少等疾病的治疗。

It tastes bitter with cold property and non-toxicity, belongs to lung, large intestine and small intestine meridian. It has the effects of clearing heat and dispelling wind, stopping bleeding and promoting diuresis. It is often used to treat dry cough and aphonia, damp-heat jaundice, hematochezia and lack of urination.

90. 火焰树

Spathodea campanulata Beauv.

火焰树是紫葳科火焰树属乔木。原产于非洲的火焰树，由于其花朵鲜艳夺目形似火焰而得名，在云南的西双版纳、广东、福建、台湾等热带或者亚热带的地区都有引种。作为药用植物，其中药名叫火焰树，火焰树的果实、根、叶都具有药用价值。

It is an arbor of Bignoniaceae and Spathodea, which is native to Africa and gained its name for its flame-like flowers. It was introduced to tropical areas, such as Xishuangbanna in Yunnan, Guangdong, Fujian, Taiwan or other or sub-hot areas. Its medicinal name is Huoyanshu and its fruits, roots and leaves have medicinal value.

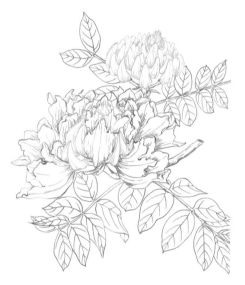

火焰树的果实具有消积止痢、活血止血的作用，主治消化不良和肠炎、痢疾等。根部具有清热凉血的作用，主治跌打损伤、筋骨疼痛、腰痛等。叶子具有清热解毒的作用，主治疮疡肿毒。

Its fruits have the effects of removing food retention and checking dysentery, promoting blood circulation and stopping bleeding, and it can be used to treat indigestion, enteritis and dysentery. Its roots have the effects of removing heat and cooling blood and can be used to treat traumatic injuries, arthralgia and myalgia, lumbago. Its leaves have the effects of clearing heat and removing toxicity and can be used to treat sore and ulcer.

91. 龙船花　　*Ixora chinensis* Lam.

龙船花是常绿小灌木茜草科龙船花属的植物，主要分布在云南、广东、广西、福建和台湾，一般多生长于树林下、灌木丛中和旷野路旁。作为药用植物，它的中药名就叫龙船花，入药部位为花朵。每年的7—10月份采收其花，将其洗净、晒干以后就可以备用，鲜品也可以使用。

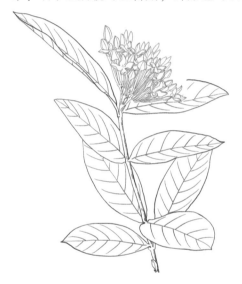

It is an evergreen shrub of rubiaceae and Ixora L., distributes in Yunnan, Guangdong, Guangxi, Fujian and Taiwan, and mainly grows under trees, in bushes and wilderness roadsides. Its medicinal name is Longchuanhua and its flowers can also be used as herbal medicine. Collect its flowers from July to October every year and they can be used as medicine after being washed clean and dried in the sun, or use its fresh flowers directly.

其味甘、淡，性凉，归肝经，具有清热凉血、散瘀止痛之功效，常用于高血压、月经不调、闭经、跌打损伤、疮疡疖肿等疾病的治疗。

It tastes sweet and bland with cold property, belongs to liver meridian. It has the effects of clearing heat and cooling blood, relieving pain by dissipating blood stasis and it is often used to treat hypertension, irregular menstruation, amenorrhea, traumatic injuries, swollen and sore of the boils.

92. 广东万年青　　　*Aglaonema modestum* Schott ex Engl.

广东万年青是天南星科广东万年青属的多年生常绿草本植物。它主要分布在我国的华南以及云南的东南部，多生长于海拔 500—1700 米的密林中。作为药用植物，其中药名叫广东万年青，入药部位是植物的根茎及叶。一般每年 10 月中下旬采挖根茎，切片晒干以后就可以备用，鲜品也可以使用；7 月中下旬采收茎叶，切断晒干以后就可以备用，鲜品也可以使用。

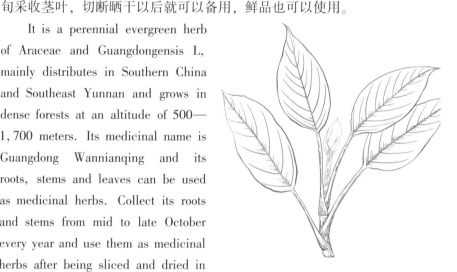

It is a perennial evergreen herb of Araceae and Guangdongensis L, mainly distributes in Southern China and Southeast Yunnan and grows in dense forests at an altitude of 500—1, 700 meters. Its medicinal name is Guangdong Wannianqing and its roots, stems and leaves can be used as medicinal herbs. Collect its roots and stems from mid to late October every year and use them as medicinal herbs after being sliced and dried in the sun, or use its fresh roots or stems directly. Leaves can be harvested in mid to late July and used as medicinal herb after being sliced and dried in the sun, or use its fresh leaves directly.

其味辛、微苦，性寒，归肺、胃、肾经，有毒，具有清热凉血、消肿拔毒、止痛的功效，用于咽喉肿痛、白喉、肺热咳嗽、吐血、热毒便血、疮疡肿毒、蛇犬咬伤等疾病的治疗。

It tastes pungent and slightly bitter with cold property and toxicity, belongs to lung, stomach and kidney meridian. It has the effects of clearing heat and cooling blood, reducing swelling and removing toxicity, relieving pain. It can be used to treat sore swollen throat, diphtheritis, cough due to lung heat, hematemesis, hematochezia, ulcer and sore skin due to pyogenic infections, snake and dog bites.

93. 散尾葵

Dypsis lutescens（H. Wendl.）Beentje & Dransf.

散尾葵是棕榈科马岛椰属丛生常绿小乔木或者灌木，也有人叫他黄椰子和凤凰尾，在滇南一带到处可见，现云南、广东、海南、广西有栽培，多植于庭园或花圃。它的叶子可以拿来做药，作为药用植物，其中药名叫散尾葵。全年都可以采收。

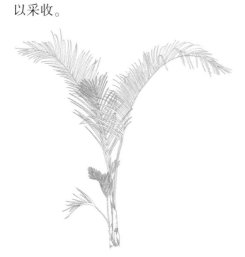

It is the evergreen arbor or shrub of palmaceae and Sacropora Genus, some people call it Huangyezi or Fenghuangwei, it can be found everywhere in Southern Yunnan and it is cultivated in gardens or flower beds in Yunnan, Guangdong, Hainan and Guangxi. The sheath fiber of its leaves can be used as medicinal herb and its medicinal name is Sanweikui, it can be collected all year round.

其味微苦、涩，性凉，归肝经，具有收敛止血的功效，常用于治疗吐血、咯血、便血、崩漏。

It tastes slightly bitter and astringent with cold property, belongs to liver meridian. It has the effect of astringing to stop bleeding and can be used to treat hematemesis, hemoptysis, hematochezia and uterine bleeding.

94. 黄花假杜鹃   *Barleria prionitis* L.

中药黄花假杜鹃为爵床科假杜鹃属植物黄花假杜鹃的根、叶或全株，在《中华本草（傣医卷）》里有详细的记载。该植物主要分布于云南西双版纳，是一味很有名的傣药。

The medicinal parts of *Huanghuajiadujuan* are its roots, leaves or whole plant of the Acanthaceae and Barleria plant, it was recorded detailedly in *Chinese Medicinal Plants（Dai Medicine）*. It is a very famous Dai medicine and mainly distributes in Xishuangbanna, Yunan province.

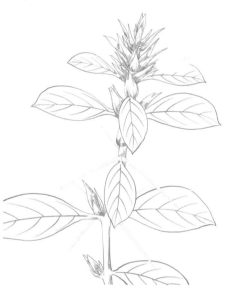

其味辛、苦，性温，具有调补水血、散瘀消肿、止痛的功效，主治体弱多病、不思饮食、跌打损伤、骨折、风寒湿痹证、肢体关节肿痛、屈伸不利、鸡眼。

It tastes pungent and bitter with warm property, and it has the effects of regulating and replenishing blood, eliminating blood stasis and removing swelling, relieving pain. It can be used to treat valetudinarianism, poor appetite, traumatic injuries, fractures, wind-cold-dampness arthralgia, swollen and painful limbs, unfavorable flexion and extension, corns.

95. 薜荔　　*Ficus pumila* L.

薜荔是一种桑科榕属常绿攀岩或匍匐的灌木植物。除云南外，主要分布于福建、江西、浙江、安徽、江苏、台湾等地。它不仅果实可以食用，其茎叶可以拿来入药。

It is an evergreen rock climbing or creeping shrub of Moraceae and Ficus genus. In addition to Yunnan, it is mainly distributed in Fujian, Jiangxi, Zhejiang, Anhui, Jiangsu and Taiwan. Not only can its fruits be edible, but its stems and leaves can also be used as herbal medicine.

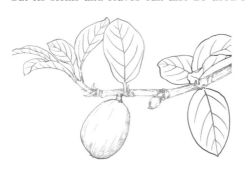

作为药用植物，其中药名叫薜荔，其味酸，性平，具有祛风、利湿、活血、解毒的功效，主治风湿痹痛、泻痢、淋病、跌打损伤、痈肿疮疖等病症。

Its medicinal name is Bili and it tastes sour with mild property. It has the effects of dispelling wind-evil, removing dampness, promoting blood circulation and detoxifying. It is mainly used to treat rheumatic arthralgia, diarrhea, gonorrhea, traumatic injuries and boils.

96. 枳实（酸橙）　　*Citrus x aurantium* L.

枳实实际上是芸香科柑橘属植物酸橙及其栽培变种或甜橙的干燥幼果。药用植物多是常绿小乔木，在长江流域或者长江以南地区都有栽培，每年 5—6 月份，将酸橙或者甜橙的幼果采收，也可以捡拾自然脱落的幼果，晒干以后就可以备用。

Zhishi is the medicinal name of dried young fruits of Citrus aurantium L. of Rutaceae and citrus or cultivar or Citrus sinensis Osbeck. Most of the medicinal plants are evergreen small arbors, cultivated in the Yangtze River basin or south of the Yangtze River, collect the young fruits of Citrus aurantium L. or Citrus sinensis Osbeck or pick up the young fruits that fall off naturally from May to June every year to use it as medicine after being dried in the sun.

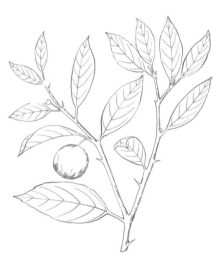

其味苦、辛、酸，性微寒，归脾、胃经，具有破气消积、化痰除痞的功效，主治胃肠积滞、湿热泻痢、胸痹、结胸、气滞胸胁疼痛、产后腹痛等病症。

It tastes bitter, pungent and sour with minor cold, belongs to spleen and stomach meridian. It has the effects of regulating Qi and removing food retention, eliminating phlegm and distention. It can be used to treat gastrointestinal stagnation and dampness-heat diarrhea, chest obstruction, chest binding, chest and hypochondrium pain due to Qi stagnation, postpartum abdominal pain.

97. 开口箭

Rohdea chinensis（Baker）N. Tanaka

开口箭是天门冬科万年青属植物，主要分布于湖南、湖北、广东及云南、陕西、安徽、浙江、江西、福建、台湾、四川等地，其中，剑叶开口箭主要分布于云南。

(Rohdea ewfolia LF. T. Wan & Tang) N. Tanuki is a plant of Asparagaceae and Rohdea, mainly distributes in Hunan, Hubei, Guangdong and Yunnan, Shaanxi, Anhui, Zhejiang, Jiangxi, Fujian, Taiwan and Sichuan, and it is mainly distributed in Yunnan.

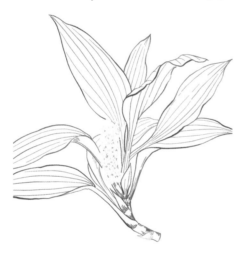

作为药用植物，它的中药名就叫开口箭。其味苦、辛，性寒，归肺、胃、肝经，有毒，具有清热解毒、祛风除湿、散瘀止痛的功效，常用于白喉，咽喉肿痛，风湿痹痛，跌打损伤，胃痛，痈肿疮毒，毒蛇、狂犬咬伤等疾病的治疗。

Its medicinal name is Kaikoujian, it has toxicity and tastes bitter and pungent with cold property, belongs to lung, stomach and liver meridian. It has the effects of clearing heat and removing toxicity, dispelling wind and eliminating dampness, relieving pain by dissipating blood stasis. It is often used to treat diphtheria, sore and swollen throat, rheumatic arthralgia, traumatic injuries, stomachache, carbuncle, bites by venomous snake and rabies.

98. 海金沙　　*Lygodium japonicum*（Thunb.）Sw.

海金沙是海金沙科海金沙属多年生攀岩草质藤本植物。海金沙多分布于西南、华东、中南及西北的陕西和甘肃等地。作为药用植物，它的中药名就叫海金沙。全草均可入药。其中干燥成熟孢子，每逢9—10月份，在孢子还未脱落的时候就采收。

It is a perennial climbing grass vine of lygodiaceae and lygodium, mainly distributes in Southwest, East China, Central and South China and Northwest Shaanxi and Gansu. etc,. Its medicinal name is Haijinsha and its whole plant as well as can be used as herbal medicine. It should be harvested before its spores falling off from September to October.

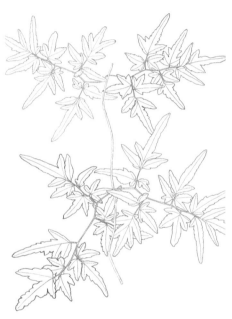

我们把地上部分叫作海金沙草，也有人把它叫作海金沙藤、金线藤、松筋草、爬山藤和鸡脚藤。每年的7—10月份将其采收，洗净晒干就可以备用。海金沙地下部分也可以入药，它的地下部分就叫作海金沙根，一般每年的8—9月份将其采挖，洗净、切片、晒干以后就可以备用。

Its above-ground parts are called Haijinshacao, or Haijinshateng, Jinxianteng, Songjincao, Pashateng and Jijiaoteng. It can be harvested from July to October and used as medicine after being washed clean and dried in the sun. In addition, its underground parts can also be used as medicine and they are called Haijinshagen, dig them out from August to September and use them as medicine after being washed clean, sliced and dried in the sun.

其味甘、咸，性寒，归膀胱、小肠经。具有清利湿热、通淋止痛的功效，主要用于尿路结石、湿疹、带下、咽喉肿痛、痄腮、水肿等疾病的治疗。

It tastes sweet and salty with cold property, belongs to bladder and small intestine meridian. It has the effects of eliminating dampness and heat, removing stone and relieving pain. It can be used to treat lithangiuria, eczema, leucorrhea, sore and swollen throat, mumps and edema.

99. 蒲桃

Syzygium jambos（L.）Alston

蒲桃为桃金娘科蒲桃属植物，人们也把它叫作水蒲桃、香果、香谷。蒲桃原产于东南亚，在我国云南、广东、广西、福建、海南、台湾、贵州都有分布。每年的 2 月就是蒲桃花开的季节，蒲桃既是美味的水果，也是我们身边的一味草药。作为药用植物，其中药名叫蒲桃，入药部位主要是植物的叶、果皮、种子及根皮。

It is the plant of myrtaceae and Syzygium Gaertn, it is called Shuiputao, Xiangguo and Xianggu. Putao is native to Southeast Asia and distributes in Yunnan, Guangdong, Guangxi, Fujian, Hainan, Taiwan and Guizhou. It blooms in February every year, and it is not only a delicious fruit, but also an herb around us. Its medicinal name is Putao and the main medicinal parts are its leaves, pericarp, seeds and root bark.

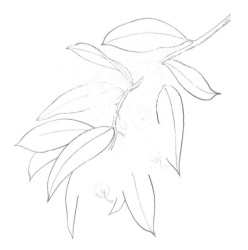

蒲桃壳：味甘、酸，性热，有暖胃健脾、补肺止嗽、破血消肿的功效，主治胃寒呃逆、脾虚泄泻、久痢、肺虚寒嗽、疝瘤。蒲桃根皮：味甘、涩，性平，无毒，凉血、收敛，主治痢疾、腹泻、刀伤出血。蒲桃叶：清热解毒，主治口舌生疮、疮疡、痘疮。蒲桃种子：健脾、止泻，主治脾虚泄泻、久痢、糖尿病。

Its shell tastes sweet and sour with hot property, and it has the effects of invigorating the spleen and warming the stomach, tonifying lung to stop cough, relieving swelling, it can be used to treat hiccup caused by stomach cold, spleen-deficiency diarrhea, chronic dysentery, lung deficiency and cold cough, tumor of abscess. Its root bark is non-toxic, tastes sweet and astringent with mild property, it has the effects of cooling blood and maintaining strength, and it can be used to treat dysentery, diarrhea, bleeding from knife wounds. Its leaves have the effects of clearing heat and removing toxicity, it can be used to treat mouth sores, sore and ulcer, variola. Its seeds have the effects of invigorating the spleen and relieving diarrhea, it can be used to treat spleen-deficiency diarrhea, chronic dysentery and diabetes.

100. 金叶子

Craibiodendron steuatum (Pierre) W. W. Sm.

金叶子是杜鹃花科金叶子属的常绿小乔木。人们又把它叫作云南金叶子、云南泡花树、云南假木荷、云南克櫑木。金叶子主要分布于云南、广西和西藏，它主要生长于海拔1200米到3200米的树林或者灌木丛中。作为药用植物，它的中药名就叫金叶子，其入药部位就是它的叶子。

Craibiodendron steuatum(Pierre) W. W. Sm. is the evergreen arbor of Ericaceae and Craibiodendron. People also call it Yunnan Jinyezi, Yunnan Paohuashu, Yunnan Jiamuhe and Yunnan Keleimu. It mainly distributes in Yunnan, Guangxi and Xizang, and grows in trees and shrubs at an altitude of 1,200 to 3,200 meters. Its medicinal name is Jinyezi and the medicinal part is its leaves.

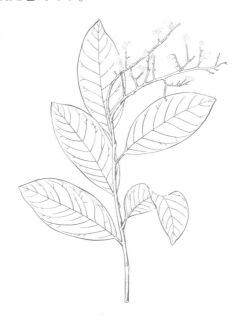

其味微辛，性温，有大毒，入肝、肾经，具有祛风活血、通络止痛的功效，主治风湿痹痛、半身不遂、跌打损伤等病症。

It has strong toxicity and tastes slight pungent with warm property, belongs to liver and kidney meridian. It has the effects of dispelling wind and promoting blood circulation, dredging collaterals and relieving pain, it can be used to treat rheumatic arthralgia, hemiplegia and traumatic injuries.

101. 叶下花(白背兔儿风)

Ainsliaea pertyoides var. *albotomentosa*
Beauverd

　　白背兔儿风，菊科兔儿风属植物，主要分布在云南、四川等地，它多生长于灌木丛或者是树林下的阴湿处。它也是一味草药，其中药名叫作叶下花，全草入药使用。叶下花，春夏两季可以采收，洁净，切段，晒干。鲜品也可以直接使用。捣细敷在患处。

It is the plant of Compositae and Ainsliaea DC, distributes in Yunan and Sichuan, mainly grows in the shade of bushes or trees. Its medicinal name is Yexiahua and its whole herbs can be used as medicinal herbs, we can collect them in Spring and Summer and use it after being cleaned, sliced and dried , or use them freshly after being mached the applied to the affectea area.

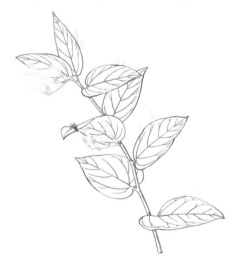

　　其味苦，性温，归肝、肾经，小毒，具有祛风除湿、散瘀止血、消肿散结的功效，用于风湿痹痛、血瘀经闭、跌打损伤、骨折肿痛、外伤出血、瘰疬结核、风寒喘咳等疾病的治疗。

It has mild toxicity and tastes bitter with warm property, belongs to liver and kidney meridian. It has the effects of dispelling wind and eliminating dampness, dispersing stasis to stop bleeding, reducing swelling and resolving mass. It can be used to treat rheumatic arthralgia, blood stasis menstrual block, traumatic injuries, fracture, traumatic bleeding, tuberculosis of scrofula, wind-cold panting and cough.

102. 朱砂草(广州蛇根草) *Ophiorrhiza cantoniensis* Hance

广州蛇根草是茜草科蛇根草属植物，为中国特有，分布于华南及西南。朱砂草，中药名，以广州蛇根草的根茎作为入药部位。每逢秋季将其采挖，洗净、晒干以后就可以备用。全草鲜品也可以直接使用。是一种主要生长于溪边、林下的草本植物。

Ophiorrhiza cantoniensis Hance is Rubiaceae and Ophiorrhiza plant, it is a kind of herb that mainly grows in the stream sides and under the forest, which is unique to China and distributed in South China and Southwest China. Its medicinal name is Zhushacao and its roots and stems of Ophiorrhiza cantoniensis Hance can be used

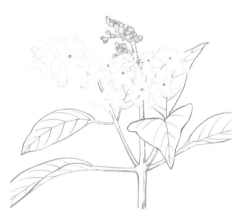

as herbal medicine. Collect them in Autumn and use them as medicine after being washed clean and dried in the sun, or use them freshly.

其味苦，性寒，归肺、脾、肝经，具有清热止咳、镇静安神、消肿止痛的功效，用于劳伤咳嗽、霍乱吐泻、神经衰弱、月经不调、跌打损伤等疾病的治疗。

It tastes bitter with cold property and belongs to lung, spleen and liver meridian, it has the effects of clearing heat and relieving cough, calming the minds and nerves, relieving swelling and pain. It can be used to treat strain cough, vomiting and diarrhea, neurasthenia, irregular menstruation and traumatic injuries.

103. 三枝叶（滇探春）

Chrysojasminum subhumile（W. W. Sm）
Banfi & Galasso

　　滇探春，俗名滇素馨，为木犀科素馨属植物。是一种原产于墨西哥的灌木或者小乔木。它一般分布于云南和四川，多生长于溪边或者是林中。三枝叶，中药名，其入药部分是滇素馨的根或叶。6—10月可以采挖其根，将其洗净、切片晒干以后就可以备用。全年可以采收其叶，切碎，鲜用或晒干。滇素馨的中药名除叫三枝叶，还叫它三岔叶、三爪皮、洗叶子。

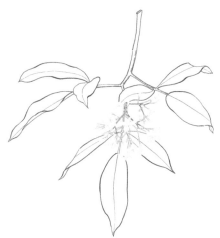

Jasminumsubhumile W. W. Smith is Oleaceae and Jasminum L. plant, it's a shrub or small arbor native to Mexico. It is commonly distributed in Yunnan and Sichuan, and grows near streams or in forests. Its medicinal name is Sanzhiye and its roots or leaves can be used as medicinal herbs, its roots can be harvested from June to October and used as herbal medicine after being washed clean, sliced and dried in the sun. Its leaves can be collected all year round and they can be used after being sliced, use them freshly or dried. In addition to the name of Sanzhiye, it is also called Sanchaye, Sanguapi and Xiyezi.

　　其味辛、微苦，性平，具有祛风除湿、止痛、止血的功效，常用于感冒发热、头痛身痛、风湿痹痛、跌打损伤、外伤出血等病症。

　　It tastes pungent and slight bitter with mild property, and it has the effects of dispelling wind evil and eliminating dampness, relieving pain and stopping bleeding. It is often used to treat cold and fever, headache and body pain, rheumatic arthralgia, traumatic injuries and traumatic bleeding.

104. 亚罗椿（浆果楝）

Cipadessa baccifera（Roth.）Miq.

浆果楝，为楝科浆果楝属植物。它主要分布于云南，多生长于海拔 500—1600 米的长绿阔叶林、疏林或者灌木丛中。它的中药名叫亚罗椿，在《全国中草药汇编》里把它叫作浆果楝秧勒，入药部分是浆果楝的根、叶。

Cipadessa baccifera(Roth.) Miq is the plant of Meliaceae and Xylocarpus, which is mainly distributed in Yunnan province and grows in long green broad-leaved forests, thin forests or bushes with an altitude of 500 to 1,600 meters. Its medicinal name is Yaluochun and it is called Jiangguo Lianqiule in *National Compilation of Chinese Herbal Medicine*, the medicinal parts are its roots and leaves.

其味苦，性凉，归肺、膀胱、小肠经，无毒，具有疏风解表、截疟的功效，常用于感冒、皮肤瘙痒、疟疾等疾病的治疗。

It is non-toxic and tastes bitter with cold property, belongs to lung, bladder and small intestine meridian. It has the effects of expelling wind evil and relieving the exterior syndrome, stopping malaria. It is often used to treat cold, skin itch and malaria.

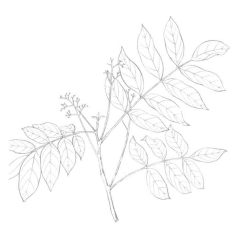

105. 针刺枣

Ziziphus mauritiana Lam.

缅枣，为鼠李科枣属植物，主要分布在云南、广东、广西、四川、福建、台湾、海南等地。作为药用植物，它的中药名就叫缅枣，又叫滇刺枣，入药部分是植物的树皮及果实。每逢秋季采收树皮，除去外皮，晒干；果实成熟后可以采收，晒干备用。

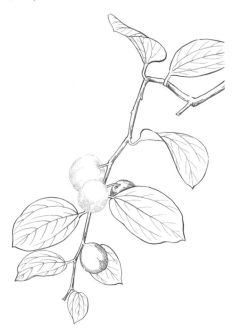

Ziziphus mauritiana Lam. is the plant of Rhamnaceae and Zizyphus and mainly distributes in Yunnan, Guangdong, Guangxi, Sichuan, Fujian, Taiwan and Hainan. Its medicinal name is Mianzao or Diancizao, its bark and fruits can be used as medicinal herbs, collect its bark every autumn and remove its skin, then dry the bark in the sun. Harvest its ripe fruits and dry them in the sun for later usage.

其味涩、微苦，性凉，具有消热止痛、收敛止泻的功效，主治烧烫伤、咽喉痛、腹泻、痢疾。

It tastes astringent and slightly bitter with cold property. It has the effects of eliminating heat and relieving pain, converging and anti-diarrhea. It is often used to treat burns and scalds, sore throat, diarrhea and dysentery.

106. 海岛棉

Gossypium barbadense L.

海岛棉，是锦葵科棉属植物，分布于云南、广东和广西等省区。作为药用植物，不仅棉花可以当中药使用，棉花子、棉花根也是我们的中药。其棉毛具有止血的功效，主治吐血、下血、血崩、金疮出血。

Gossypium barbadense L. is the plant of Malvaceae and Gossypium and distributes in Yunnan, Guangdong and Guangxi. Its flowers, seeds and roots can be used as medicinal herbs. It is a good herbal medicine, its cotton wool has the effect of stopping bleeding and it is mainly used to treat vomiting blood, hematochezia, metrorrhagia and incised wound bleeding.

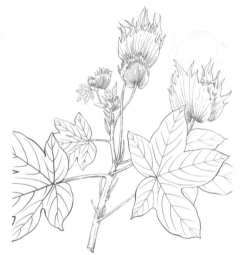

107. 蛇葡萄

Ampelopsis glandulosa（Wall.）Momiy.

蛇葡萄，是葡萄科蛇葡萄属的木质藤本植物。云南人又叫它野葡萄、山葡萄、爬山虎、过江龙。它在长江以南的大部分地区都有分布，多生长于海拔 300—1200 米的山谷树林，或灌木丛中。作为药用植物，它的中药名就叫蛇葡萄，其茎叶是可以入药的，一般 7—9 月份采收，洗净、晒干以后备用，鲜品也可以使用。

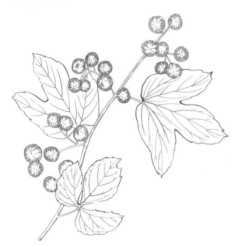

Ampelopsis glandulosa（Wall.）Momiy. is the woody vine plant of Vitaceae and Ampelopsis, Yunnan people also call it Yeputao, Shanputao, Pashanhu and Guojianglong. It is mostly distributed in the areas of the South of the Yangtze River and grows in the valley forests or bushes with an altitude of 300 to 1, 200 meters. Its medicinal name is Sheputao and its stems and leaves can be used as herbal medicine. Harvest its stems and leaves from July to September and use them as herbal medicine after being washed clean and dried in the sun, or we can use it fresh stems and leaves directly.

其味辛、苦，性凉，具有清热解毒、祛风活络、止痛、止血、敛疮的功效，常用于风湿性关节炎、呕吐、腹泻、溃疡、跌打损伤肿痛、疮疡肿毒、外伤出血、烧烫伤等病症的治疗。

It tastes pungent and bitter with cold property. It has the effects of clearing heat and removing toxicity, dispelling wind evil and activating collaterals, relieving pain, stopping bleeding and healing sore. It is commonly used to treat rheumatic arthritis, vomiting, diarrhea, ulcers, traumatic injuries, sore and ulcer, traumatic bleeding, burns and scalds.